The Beginning

Like so many stories, this tale began long ago on another fall day when life for our family was very different. It was a beautiful, crisp blue sky day that I spent walking along the lake with my younger brother, enjoying the fresh air and sharing the treasured secrets on our hearts. He was struggling with alcohol addiction and working his way through treatment. I struggled with ten years of dashed dreams trying to conceive a child. Years before my parents had faced the reality of the pain and confusion drinking caused in our family, and began renewal and restoration. My brother still felt the aftermath of those years and his statement burned in my heart *"Jodee, doesn't it make you angry at God that you can't have a child? After all, there were times it felt like you raised us."* I didn't want to be childless, but my husband and I didn't feel we could make the life changes necessary to adopt an older child after fostering several children.

My heart ached as I drove home and I prayed my first sincere prayer. *"Lord, send me to speak where and when you desire. My fertility and this child issue are yours."* Finishing this short prayer I felt refreshed. I closed the door on barrenness, handed my fertility over to the Father and drove home under happy puffy purple and pink clouds toward a golden sunset.

I left my grief in more capable hands than mine.

Our lives during that time were busy. My business was flourishing. I was chosen Entrepreneur of the Year in 1986 by the International Council of Small Business and speaking internationally on business entrepreneurship. Our design studio had won Best of Show in national competition. My clients were happy. Life was exciting and Karl and I were free to go and do just what we willed.

All this was about to change with one phone call.

you can not see my disability on the outside.

I like to make myself look pretty and I like to wear cool clothes like the other kids. people seem to notice me and I stand out in a crowd. I laugh loudly, walk loudly and talk loudly. I like a good time.

Individuals with prenatal alcohol exposure often look like everyone else. The facial differences attributed to Fetal Alcohol Syndrome (FAS) occur during only two days of gestation, so most persons affected have hidden physical and neurological differences. Their actions and reactions to life experiences are often misunderstood.

They often have problems receiving, processing, storing and utilizing information due to neurological dysfunction.

Prenatal Alcohol Exposure is 100% preventable.

How do we go on? The same way we get back on a bike when we fall, or back on a horse when we are thrown! The same way we shove one more mouthful of carrots into the mouth of a baby that is sure to spit most of it out. We know that some little part containing nourishment will stay in that reluctant little mouth! Most of all, we try to realize that every moment spent with our children helps them learn, helps them achieve, helps them know we are on their team. And then we look at our child's wonderful face and start planning tomorrow!

Lisa, FASD Mom

Mothering begins at conception, not at birth.
Ann Streissguth, Ph.D.

"Mrs. Kulp, we have a four-and-one-half month old, dying baby girl.
We need a licensed foster family to consider a high-risk legal adoption.
If you are interested, we will need you to fill out adoption papers."

Twelve hours after my first sincere prayer, my new life began to unfold. We hadn't filled out papers to become adoptive parents. Regardless, we were getting a child – a baby, a dying baby girl. Liz would soon join our family and life would never be the same. Who would say 'no' after ten years of waiting for a child? I decided the door to parenting a child was being flung open. The Lord had answered my prayer in his wonderful Kingly way and, as adoption and babies often do, everything felt very magical. My baby, our baby was in my arms.

At that moment, my husband and I believed that love, consistency and stability changes everything. So, we poured everything we had into this special little person to undo all the damage that had been done. We didn't know how wrong we were. But we soon found out. ***All the love in the world can't undo the hidden damage done by alcohol to the brain and body of a small unborn child.*** It would be twelve and a half years before we got a diagnosis of Fetal Alcohol Effects (FAE).

Persons exposed to alcohol before birth inherit lifelong brain damage – a 100% preventable legacy. FASD is not curable. They are a medical diagnosis. A child does not 'grow out of it.' It manifests itself differently in each person as the alcohol attacks the tiny growing child through the bloodstream of the mother. It randomly damages many systems in the brain and/or body. The deformities for many individuals with FASD are hidden from view, making this disability even more devastating to those who live with it daily. Most persons with FASD look like the average person. Many are beautiful and some have high IQs. Researchers have not been able to come up with a one-size-fits-all diagnosis or treatment of prenatal alcohol exposure. We are only at the beginning stages of public awareness. There is much work to be done. Liz and I hope this book, *The Best I Can Be: Living With Fetal Alcohol Syndrome/ Effects,* can contribute to this work.

I'm not angry my birth mom drinking when I was in her stomach. She didn't know She was hurting me.

I am adopted and my mom died so no one will ever know when or how much or how often my mom drank. I just know it affected me and I have to live with it.

TRY THIS:

Break a raw egg into a wine glass.
Add one ounce of alcohol.
Watch the clear part develop white streaks as the alcohol 'cooks' it.

Imagine these are a baby's dead and damaged cells from alcohol.

Imagine being deluged in a sea of alcohol unable to escape.

Just imagine.

Both the mother and the child are victims of alcohol. The biological mother did not knowingly harm the unborn child. As the adoptive, foster or biological mother you must move beyond shame, guilt or anger in order to help your child and yourself.

FASD mom

While most infants are devouring information from the world around them and making neuron connections, infants exposed to drugs and/or alcohol may be going through months of withdrawal — inability to feed, high-pitched inconsolable cries, light sensitivity, and an aversion to touch.

Jon (FASD) loves to shovel snow or dirt for the neighbors. He volunteers to bring in the garbage can or fetch things from the basement.

Bev, FASD mom

What a tangled web we enter when we cross over denial into the maze of alcohol and prenatal exposure! I truly believed I left alcohol abuse behind when I began my adult life. Yet, looking back, at least five of the foster children placed in my husband and my care exhibited behaviors related to prenatal alcohol exposure. And, even though I had consumed only limited amounts of alcohol over the last 25 years, there were at least five occasions when I could have damaged an unborn child if I was pregnant. As Jesus said to the men asking for the woman to be stoned for adultery, *"Let him who has not sinned cast the first stone."* All of us, whether we have chosen to imbibe alcohol or not, need to drop our stones and walk away just as those men did 2,000 years ago.

Public understanding of prenatal alcohol exposure is beginning, and it is commonly thought FASD happens only to the babies of poor, undereducated women. Not true! It is not only alcoholic mothers who bear prenatally exposed children. In today's western society the mothers most at risk enjoy higher household incomes, are college educated and have careers. One bout of excessive 'binge' drinking is damaging. The damage occurs in specific cells that are developing that day. Just as there are many different types of drinkers, so are there various kinds of physical and neurological damage to cells of unborn children resulting from drinking. For these children – the damage is done – there is no undo button.

This is conceivable once you understand that 1.5 oz. of liquor, 12 oz. of beer, 12 oz. of wine cooler and 5 oz. of wine all contain similar amounts of alcohol. And this alcohol in the body of the unborn baby is seven times as volatile as in an adult. What begins as relaxation for the mother deluges the child. No longer will that child enjoy the life given as a gift at conception.

Life for families of children with FASD becomes a complex maze of isolation, misunderstanding, and twenty-four hour a day care with little or no breaks. Thankfully, skillful parenting, a stable and structured home environment, early diagnosis, public awareness, intensive and appropriate intervention can make an enormous difference in the prognosis for the child. ***Let Liz and me take you on our journey inside FASD.***

When I first came home as a foster baby I would not look at people or let anyone touch me.

Mom says she put me in a Snuggle Sack under her big shirt so I could experience our family and relax. She said I was stiff like a board and shake.

It didn't take us long to realize that this was a special child and regular parenting strategies were not going to be effective.

Parenting our daughter meant we had to seek insights beyond the ordinary parenting books. Many times we felt inadequate and we learned to draw wisdom from each other.

We learned to listen to our hearts, work together as a team and then use our heads to discover her needs.

People who suffer from addictions do suffer. It is a lifelong battle. You don't just stop and get on with life. You struggle daily with yourself, with booze, and with others who might hurt you without even knowing it. We (alcoholics) are very much like the child with FASD. Our thoughts and actions are not always reasonable, but we can learn to change... slowly. The key for me is that I live my life one day at a time — and on really bad days — one minute at a time.

I have had to rebuild my life. I have had to learn to trust. I have lost friends because of my anger. I am beginning, just beginning, to learn how to heal the hurting child within me. I am beginning to feel better.

Biolclyde, FASD mom

What Kinds of Damage Can Occur From Alcohol In Utero Exposure?

Primary disabilities attributed to prenatal alcohol exposure
(Possible disabilities a child may be born with)

- Death
- Heart failure
- Heart defects
- Renal (liver) failure
- Height and weight deficiencies
- Asthma
- Immune system malfunctioning
- Mental retardation
- Developmental delay
- Developmental speech and language disorder
- Developmental coordination disorder
- Tremors
- Tourette's traits
- Autistic traits

- Deafness
- Central auditory processing disorder
- Loss of intellectual functioning (IQ)
- Little or no retained memory
- Severe loss of intellectual potential
- ADD/ADHD Attention deficit disorders
- Extreme impulsiveness
- Cerebral palsy
- Tight hamstrings
- Rigidity

- Complex seizure disorder
- Epilepsy
- Mild to severe vision problems
- Dyslexia
- Adaptive esotropia (cross-eyed)
- Serious maxilo-facial deformities
- Cleft palate
- Dental abnormalities
- Sensory Integration
- Hyper sensitivity
- Night terrors

- Sleep disorder
- Precocious puberty
- Sociopathic behavior
- Poor judgment
- Cognitive perseveration
- Higher than normal to dangerously high pain tolerance
- Little or no capacity for interpersonal empathy
- Little or no capacity for moral judgment
- Echolalia (repeat words sans understanding)

Sources: Malbin, Streissguth, Morse, Ritchie

And I have to live with it

I discovered embryology was not a subject to which a great deal of attention was given in medical school. This made me wonder if perhaps many unsolved medical mysteries had their roots in this period of greatest learning, most rapid growth, and greatest vulnerability. When the body is first learning how to be a body and the brain is learning the vast majority of what it will know about being a brain.

Julie Motz (1998)

Secondary disabilities
(May developed as a result of failure to properly deal with the primary disabilities.)

- **Education**
  - Learning difficulties
  - Disruptive
  - Disrespective
  - Poor relationships
  - Chemical use
  - Disobedience
  - Dropping out
  - Expulsions
  - Suspensions
- **Confinement**
  - Jail
  - Mental health

- – Alcohol or drug treatment
- **Mental Health**
  - Depression
  - Anxiety
  - Attachment
  - Eating disorders
  - ADHD/ADD
  - Hallucinations
  - Mental illness
  - Suicide
- **Independence**
  - Social problems

- – Poor peer choices
- – Victimization
- – Addiction/Alcoholism
- – Behavioral problems
- – Reactive outbursts
- – Chronic job issues
- – Conduct
- – Poverty/Homelessness
- **Sexuality**
  - Promiscuity
  - Prostitution
  - Inappropriate touching or advances

- – Voyeurism
- – Obscene phone calls
- – Compulsions
- – Early pregnancy
- – Sexual acting out
- **Legal**
  - Run away
  - Delinquency
  - Violence / Theft
  - Property crimes
  - Sexual misconduct

Most sorrowfully, we found that the combination of their superficially good verbal skills and their behavior problems made them unacceptable candidates for most traditional treatment programs. The girls were often teenage mothers, the boys in trouble with the law... *Ann Striessguth, Ph.D.*

When I was a baby I cried alot and mom and dad had a nurse help them. her name was nancy.

I could not go into the store without getting very scared and angry

I didnot like to be near a lot of people or noise or bright lights. I would sit in the Shopping cart and Shake until I Started Screaming.

Bright light, intense smells and loud noises may overload the brain. Children may squint or cover their eyes in bright light (sun, snow, fluorescent), put their hands to their ears to block out noise (blenders, cars, vacuum cleaners), or scream because of unpleasant smells.

I had never experienced a child as intense or volatile as my baby. Fortunately, we had a registered nurse to help us. It took a tag team of three adults to meet her needs.

A child whose body is hypersensitive to touch will actually feel discomfort from touch and stiffen or pull away from hugs.

Toni Hager

www.kidscanlearn.net

I don't think many people, including specialists know what FASD is. For me and my husband, it was a 'revelation' when we read about FASD and recognized and under- stood some of the strange behavior of our children

Gosia, FASD mom

Liz was unable to tolerate normal infant formula, so we worked with a clinical nutritionist to develop a nutrition program to meet her needs. Our family diet changed to permit Liz to grow.

Jodee, FASD mom

Two big brown eyes lay sullenly within a placid little face. Those two big eyes looked neither left nor right and were unable to focus or connect with another human being. Multiple moves in the child protection system provided her enough experience to know that love hurts and humans can't be trusted. At less than eleven pounds and five-months-old, Liz decided life was too hard, she was quitting. The medical profession calls it failure-to-thrive.

I held my new infant with the incredible love of one who had longed ten years for a child. This wasn't a cuddly baby. She bristled. Her body straightened into an unbending board. Her mouth opened and her eyes closed. We were awash in our first neurological and emotional explosion. I insisted on holding her – she resisted. We compromised by settling her into life under my large sweatshirt, riding against my bare skin in a snuggle sack. The sweatshirt provided the security she needed to experience life in our family without feeling like it was assaulting her senses. Over time she acclimated to the sounds and sensations of our home, the warmth and smells of my body, and began to accept some caregiving touch. We adapted to sleepless nights, screaming, and baby messes. She settled into rocking, singing, massages and warm baths on Mom's stomach.

Baby books would be worthless in parenting this special child.
We would need to parent from our hearts. We prayed for help and wisdom.

Help in parenting Liz came in remarkable ways. Our new neighbor was a registered nurse needing immediate income. She had raised five children of her own, and had the patience of a saint. Liz slept for less than two hours at a time, was a projectile vomiter, hated touch, was unattached to humans, and cried for hours. She needed more care than either my husband or I could provide.

Having been foster parents, we knew that keeping the adults healthy physically, mentally and emotionally was vital when working with complex children. So I returned to work part-time for my own respite, and Nancy cared for Liz. Liz grew and began thriving under the constant intense attention and stimulation of three adult caregivers. Four weeks after she arrived in our home, at six months, she made eye contact. I rejoiced! There was a spirit in this child and together we'd help it grow. Liz's will to live emerged and we sailed on an uncharted ocean.

I didn't like seams in clothes or socks so I would wear them inside out. I didn't like to change clothes in the morning so I would change clothes at night and sleep in them.

I didn't like my hair combed or touched, but I liked my back scratched.

The core problem neurological damage needs to be recognized, otherwise persons with FASD are subjected to unreasonably high expectations and experience chronic failure when they don't respond to traditional therapy or are unable to learn to behave.

Teresa Kellerman
www.fasstars.com

Living with sensory integration issues is difficult for both the child and the family. Overstimulation and/or understimulation is common with children who have been prenatally exposed to alcohol.

Everyday things become big things:
- **looking at a person and sucking on a bottle at the same time**
- **clothing and shoes**
- **smells in environment**
- **daily grooming issues for hair and skin**
- **groups of people or family gatherings**
- **the sun, the wind or the rain**
- **loud or sudden noises**
- **inappropriate pain responses**
- **too soft, too hard, too cold, too hot!**

As a school psychologist I often felt I was in the twilight zone, having to pick out one processing disorder over another as the main problem. In reality a whole raft of issues contributes to learning difficulties — social problems, auditory processing, memory, abstraction and organization issues. It would be much easier to call the whole thing neurological dysfunction with these features. And then look individually at each feature.   Kathy

I envision that someday prenatal exposure to alcohol of our children will be a thing of the past. Until that time, our children, their families and society will have to learn to live with the complexities of FASD. Early in my understanding, I dreamt that my daughter and I were trying to get into our car to go home, but huge alligators blocked our path. Finally, just as I awoke, an alligator grabbed my finger.

As I shared my dream with a friend, she advised me, *"Those alligators are real and are after our lives and our kids' lives. You know what? Let the alligators have that finger! It is our job to protect our kids and help them find a safe passage."* In essence that is what Liz and I are doing by writing this book, giving those chomping, biting, ferocious alligators our fingers in writing and getting on with loving and living our lives. We hope within these pages we begin to provide a language of understanding so that other families can find what they need to build bridges toward safe passages.

Living with prenatal alcohol exposure is difficult for everyone. The person exposed prenatally to alcohol may be impulsive, have limited cause-and-effect reasoning, have memory and processing issues, have difficulty understanding abstract ideas, have trouble with money, time and math, get easily frustrated, and be volatile.

Imagine you are in a foreign land and do not know the language. How effectively can you run your life?

Faced with this set of day-to-day behaviors, many people unknowingly label the person as 'bad' instead of neurologically injured and physically inefficient. All the therapy in the world isn't going to make the brain damage disappear and misplaced treatment can increase the secondary disabilities parents work so hard to avoid. People tend to put 'normal' interpretations on FASD behavior, which makes the individual with FASD appear to be manipulative, controlling, vengeful, etc. A normal person may be able to put that much thought into something and be controlling or manipulative, but a person with FASD behavior is usually innocent impulse without restraint. Professionals not intending to inflict harm may consider parents who are providing the best parenting they are capable of to be bad parents. The child would be a 'better' child with 'proper' parenting. Some professionals are like the five blind men trying to describe an elephant. One says, *"The elephant is a long and flexible animal."* The other says, *"No, he is a round tall, animal."* Another says, *"No, he is hairy and bristly."* Another says *"He is heavy, smooth and pointy."* And the last one says *"He is flat and can fly."* Being the parent standing under the rear end of the elephant, I observe they are all wrong – FASD is much more complex and encompassing. You never really know when you are going to get dumped on.

Students find more FASD Information: *www.fasteen.com*

The sun really bothered my eyes.
I did't like anything too hot or too cold. We live in Minnesota and it can be too hot in the Summer and to cold in the winter.
I donot like any changes I would wear my bathing suit in the winter. and winter coat in the Summer.

Sensitivity to glare, brightness and intensity of various lighting conditions including sunlight, incandescent and fluorescent lighting may be intolerable. Black and white contrast in text may make characters unreadable. Letters, numbers and musical notes may vibrate, shift, move and/or disappear.

Reactions include discomfort and difficulty concentrating. Problems with spatial relationships may occur in getting on and off escalators, running and stopping, going up and down stairs, or balancing on a tile floor.

Traveling in a car with Liz was difficult. The sun bothered her eyes and she squished up her little face screaming, "Eyes, eyes." In stores she covered her head with her blanket to avoid colors, lights, people and noise.

Jodee, FASD mom

Just because a person cannot love you as you desire doesn't mean that person is not loving you with all the love they have to give.

I thought we were adopting a healthy, little baby. I felt so betrayed.

FASD dad

You cannot defend yourself and grow at the same time, either on the cellular or the body level. Your energy can be focused only on one of these functions at a time.

Julie Motz (1998

HANGING ON FOR DEAR LIFE

Four multiple caregivers within five months, despite their love and competency, were devastating to Liz's healthy infant development. A young child can accommodate some shifting, but eventually the child gives up, suffering profound emotional and developmental loss. These issues of development and attachment further complicated the already difficult life Liz faced after conception. Still, my husband and I believed that good medical care, consistent daily schedules, one-on-one stimulation, and constant loving caregivers could meet Liz's needs.

Environment continued to be a huge battleground. Liz was tactile defensive which means she was hypersensitive to touch, light, sound, smells and movement. Even at age seven, if we touched, brushed up against her or physically directed her to safety, she screamed, *"Owie you're hurting me. Stop hurting me."* How could normal loving touches feel painful to her? Why did she shove or push us away? Only her beloved blanket *'Gee'* protected her and she securely bundled herself to settle into our laps for comfort, songs, stories and reading.

Her favorite early childhood outfit was a diaper or panties. Her preferred hairstyle was unwashed and unkempt. We chose clothes based on softness, flexibility and comfort. We removed labels and turned clothes inside out. We avoided cuffs and elastic and devised alternatives for mittens and boots by using Daddy's big warm woolen socks over velcro strapped shoes. It made no sense to fight with laces. We found a soft, warm, fuzzy rabbit fur hat to keep little ears from freezing.

At each turn in our FASD journey we encountered rough terrain where we needed to build bridges and make detours to create a semi-normal life. Crowded spaces, elevators, standing in line, tents or the backseat of the car enclosed her and she felt crushed. Sunlight glistening off the snow or fluttering through the trees overstimulated her eyes. Loud noises and background conversation caused her to cover her ears. Overwhelmed meant overreaction and we learned when we managed Liz's environment we enjoyed a bright eyed, happy child.

We exposed her to new and varied experiences in small bits knowing someday she must learn to live in the chaos of the adult world and still enjoy life. My dreams of library visits, children's museums, art fairs and circuses were replaced with a romper room of homebased stimulation.

When I was a little child I didn't to be touched, So mom made up sign language Stories using our fingers.

I didn't like hugs or kisses. I ran and hugged mom first when I was 10. Mom went into the window and broke it

I learned to hug when I was 12. Now I like Hugs.

I invented finger play stories so I could wiggle her toes, rub her back, arms and legs and touch her face and hands. The Teddy Bear Garden and Little Turtle were two of her favorites.

We spent hours writing letters and numbers on her back guessing the secret message mom was writing.

These games allowed us to begin to touch Liz in a variety of healthy ways.

Some children with FASD may seek out inappropriate or excessive touch.

Liz often held her hands in tightly closed fists. I would stroke the top of her hand and tell her her hand looked like a little turtle. I would ask the turtle if I could take a journey to find her sister turtle who lived on the other side of her noggin.'She would always nod her head 'yes', and I would slowly march my fingers zigzag up her arm, find her elbow and ask if I still had permission to find the sister turtle. The climb over the shoulders and up the neck to the head was always treacherous and we would lightly march around her mouth, nose, ears and closed eyes asking each if we could visit. Then we would journey down her other arm. At the bottom, the little turtle (her thumb) would pop out, she would smile and I could hug the whole child!

OVERSTIMULATION – SHOPPING TIL LIZ POPPED

As a person with tactile defensiveness, Liz is very sensitive to random movement. She told us stores, schools and clinics made her head crazy. More than once I left a full shopping cart to attend to the more important needs of my child. One minute she was calm and smiling. The next minute she exploded into an episode of uncontrolled screaming. These were limbic rages and not temper tantrum.

We practiced movement with wooden wagon rides, packed with her blankie 'Gee', her beloved little brother David and three harnessed wonder doggies. When she felt life was getting overstimulating, we taught her to stop, close her eyes and say *"Stop, Focus, Control."* One day in the store, two-year-old Liz held onto the shopping cart, her body shaking, eyes squeezed tight, fists clenched, shouting *"Control me! Control me! Me control me!"* Store patrons walked quickly past glaring at me. The difference in our understanding of the situation was chasms apart – I, proud of my darling daughter working so hard to cope with sensory issues, the public debating whether to be a judge and the jury. We quickly checked out.

Liz's response behavior is magnified ten-fold compared with most other children. We called it accelerated normal. It may not be unusual for a child to take free colorful chocolate suckers and stick them in her underwear to free hands for other experiences. The FASD highlights came into play after the chocolate melted in the underwear into a gooey mess and my tactile defensive child hated this feeling. It became magnified to horrific proportions when Mom added cool water to the goo in a public washroom and it hardened pulling her skin tight. I expected social service sirens for our public nuclear meltdown.

It was twelve years before we understood the roots of her dilemmas, the cause of anxiety in school and her store headaches. We didn't know that Liz felt and heard fluorescent lights buzz. They made her world dance and she tried to avoid them. In our home we switched to 'full spectrum' flourescents which were significantly less troublesome for her. Liz learn to be assertive in clinic and group environments regarding her lighting needs and even today she may wear sunglasses to the dental office or colored contact lenses to dim the light. We worked with a developmental optometrist and neurodevelopmentalist who taught us eye exercises to help Liz's eyes function better with various common lighting. With the correct therapy at thirteen, she no longer flipped out and popped in the store. She shopped.

Family parties too noisy and busy.

I would add more noise and get busy to. It felt like I was a wind up toy, dad would say "who put a quarter in you?"

When we went to family parties mom and I would go little hiding corner to be alone.

We arrived late and left early . . .

We practiced STOP.
Stand still.
Think.
Observe.
Protect yourself.

We prepared for holidays and special occasions in advance by role playing and practicing in our playroom.

We advised our friends and relatives of our child's specific needs.

Crowds and large gatherings cause a lot of stress. I have a hard time mingling and fitting in. I feel awkward, like a lost needle in a haystack, overwhelmed with nothing to say. Put me with 3 or 4 people I'm "OK." I can interact and share. I've been this way all my life. I still believe I don't have much to offer to the conversation!

Steve
FASD, 43 years old

Liz wants to behave like other children. She cannot see beyond the moment or past a situation. She reacts 'out-of-control' — the only way she is capable of, when stressed or overloaded. After she has had time to calm down and regroup, I provide her with new ways of coping and we role play.

Jodee, FASD mom

FAMILY GATHERINGS

Large family gatherings, relatives visiting or friends over for dinner overstimulated Liz. The traditions we embraced with fondness sent Liz into a tailspin — disrupting the security of her routine. Projects and celebrations we rejoiced in exhausted her. Her surrounding environment was steeped in distractions. People she didn't know or recognize expected her to react like other children.

I tried to imagine what it must be like. I sat on the floor with my eyes closed, trying to listen to all twelve conversations at one time, feeling very small and overwhelmed. My child was a stranger in a strange land, unable to separate languages or sequence change.

The electrical storms in Liz's brain caused meltdowns. These rages are often misinterpreted as willful disobedience or temper tantrums. In reality, the person with FASD has little or no control over the experience once it begins. The surrounding audience's best defense is keeping the individual safe and minimizing the destructive forces of the tornado within. After a rage, Liz had no idea regarding her behavior. She was sweet as could be. Onlookers remained stunned while my heart pumped loudly. Verbal escalation on our part or physical restraint of Liz increased the duration of the rage and we learned to move her into a safe, quiet space and monitor. If we could not move her we talked to her softly and encouraged eye contact. To others it appeared like complete marshmallow appeasement and they believed her behavior to be our fault. They believed we lost control when in reality we were maintaining control. As Diane Malbin so rightly stated, we needed to parent differently not harder. Karl and I questioned how many abused children are also prenatally affected.

We found ourselves dodging friends and family. We hid in out-of-the-way nooks and crannies in their homes to soften the stimulation and yet experience the feasts and celebrations. We dined under a table peering out beneath the table cloth. We ate our dinner in the quietness of a bathroom, enjoying fine dining on a furry toilet seat cover. Many times we huddled in the coat room listening to muffled conversations, wrapped in our blanket friend 'Gee', while Liz regrouped. I sang softly the songs of the season. In the homes of our dearest friends, Liz sometimes took a hot bath and snuggled sleepily in my arms. Finally, Mom enjoyed evenings of adult conversation, something very rare during the early days of raising Liz.

Mom would sing and rock me and teel stories before bed. I had night terrors and I would run through the house Screaming and crying and talking.

I would take warm bubbly baths before bed to help me go to Sleep. Mom would use the drying machine to get me dry.

Imagine you are sitting in a very hard chair that is too small for you so your body is compressed. The floor is moving ever so slightly. The lights in the room are flashing. There is a ringing alarm clock and a humming sound that seems to never end. Your friend is talking to you but you only are able to understand every third or fourth word. Then your dog jumps upon you with kisses after being sprayed by skunk.

Now imagine you have no control over any of this. You cannot get away. People are moving and talking faster and faster and faster. **Imagine.**

Liz often awoke disoriented and screamed for 45 minutes after she napped. Once she regrouped, she would hop off my lap, smile, run and play as if nothing happened. I was left behind exhausted.

Nancy, Liz's RN Nurse

Keeping Liz safe at night was a concern. She often awoke from a deep sleep screaming. Then she walked through the house terrorized, shaking and crying followed by our beloved doggies. We would comfort her and direct her back to safety. She never remembered the experience. Once on vacation she escaped from our condo and walked into a nearby condo, her parents fast on her heels. Our door had been locked.

Jodee, FASD mom

PICKING OUR BATTLES

Transition time for a person with FASD is often very difficult. A change in routine can send them over the edge. Any situation could become a battle if we placed normal expectations on Liz. Bedtimes and morning times were especially trying. Changing clothes topped her list of frustrations. Jammies after baths were impossible. We developed gentle bedtime rituals to help limit her night terrors. We said

She would wrap me in a big towel and rub me really hard. The hard rubbing felt warm. Then I would let her dry my hair.

good night to the day with a warm bath and wrapped her in a soft terry towel. I rubbed her tiny body dry, and she settled enough to let me dry and brush her frazzled hair while I sang children's songs. We rolled her in ' Gee' and piled covers on top of her. In the corner of her bedroom tiny Christmas tree lights twinkled. We snuggled together reading and retelling daily adventures to reinforce what she had learned. She slept in her most comfortable jammies — her blanket 'Gee.' Eventually she fell asleep, but never for long.

I heard Liz's ear-piercing scream as I lifted a shovelful of three-foot deep snow after a Minnesota blizzard. Liz flew out the door and through the air as she frantically looked for us. Her naked body landed neck deep in the snow. At bedtime we told her to go to the window and wave to us when she awoke. She didn't remember and felt abandoned. For two hours she cried. She shed tears beginning a deeper attachment to her family. The door to five previous abandonments opened. She was developed enough to attach words to feelings. She was almost seven-years-old.

Liz has always been a problem solver of unique solutions. She wore her next day's outfit to bed from that point on to avoid the morning clothes transition. It took until age thirteen before a pair of flannel trousers and a big polar fleece shirt served as pajamas. It took until later in her teen years before she enjoyed picking out morning clothes.

FASD families need to be creative and flexible in the little daily issues. Some families adjust by making the form of a person on the floor with the child's clothes before going to bed. The child just jumps into them upon arising. Others heat clothes in the dryer and challenge the children to jump in before they get cold.

Mom and Nancy read me hundreds of stories. We did lots art and puzzies. They taught me to count but I told them they didn't know the right way. It was 1.2.3.5.6.7.9.10 For you for me is not a number and I ate my dinner.

Everyone thought I was smart. I knew 60 breeds of dogs when I was three and all my colors when I was two. I knew all the words to songs and sang all the time.

Over time we got past most of the attachment issues.

Yet there were many missing pieces – teaching her was very, very difficult. It was like filling a bucket full of holes. As fast as the information went in, it seemed to pour out.

She couldn't cut, hop, skip or do many of the things the other children were doing and I couldn't figure out how to teach her.

When Liz was three, we had three loving standard poodles, each with very different person alities. Abraham, our jet black male, had just absconded with something he thought was delightful. My husband caught him and stated, "That dog needs jail!"

"Daddy, what doe Isak need?" Liz asked.

"Well, Isak needs consistent parenting or he gets into trouble."

"What does Joey need?" she continued.

"Joey just needs love, he always wants to b good. What kind of parenting do you need Liz?"

"I need attention parenting!" she loudly declared.

Jodee, FASD mo

Remember you are a super parent. You are ju too tired to notice it.

ANIMALS PAVED THE WAY TO AFFECTION

Animals are a large part of our family life. We instill in our family members the need to care deeply for all creatures using gentleness, consideration and kindness; tempered with structure, rules and obedience. We've trained some wonderful animals – lovingly, kindly and inventively. I was not surprised when my dear friend Liv said, *"Jod, if you can get through to those animals...you can reach Liz."*

We hand-raised tiny wild baby bunnies and returned them grown to the Owl Forest. We watched scoops of tadpoles grow into frogs in our kitchen and then sadly jump into Sunday morning orange juice. Birds built their nests outside our school window. A friendly Siamese Fighting Beta fish swam in a lighted tank to protect children needing to use the toilet in the night. Liz raised baby chicks and ducklings that sweetly perched on her shoulders. Two african frogs lived in Liz's room for five years!

Age ten is when most children move from concrete to abstract academics. For children with FASD who often never acquire abstraction this change in their school and peer relationships is devastating. Stuck in earlier child thinking and playing, their friends move on in new interests of study, play and humor. It is the beginning of a new loneliness. Our friend Greg, of Critters and Company was given an abused cockatiel who had been evicted from five homes due to obnoxious bird behavior. Feisty 'Emily' reminded Greg of Liz. After he cleared it with Karl and me, he talked Liz into taking the bird on as a challenge. He explained to her that the bird had behaviors he saw in her – hissing, biting, jumping up and down, and squawking. Since she knew how it felt to have those behaviors, perhaps she could help the bird behave better. It was her job to help the bird become a better bird. Liz's new title was 'Animal Trainer.' Our new parenting job was to protect the bird.

One day I watched in amazement as a yellow-feathered, eight-inch bird and a frustrated girl jumped up and down, hissed, spat, squawked and screamed at each other, neither of them budging from her own vantage point. The scene was comical and I thought *"Dear God, is that how I look to You when I yell at Liz?"*

Over time, the bird and the girl became loving to each other. Liz wanted the bird to allow her to touch it. This desire allowed us to share how we also felt when she didn't want us to touch her. Soon after, Liz told me she loved me. Shortly after, she hugged her father for the first time. He had waited ten long years.

I memorized the alphabet song but couldn't put it together. The letters kept dancing on the paper.

Why wasn't b,d,p,q all the same. They looked the same to me. So did w,m, and 3,7, and 6 and 9,5 and 2. I didn't know why you had to read one way left to right when you could read right to left too. I still have trouble knowing right and left sometimes.

Liz's wisdom often startles me with its logical clarity. It would be much easier if we could see her unusual circuitry.

To Liz, the letters b, d, p and q were all the same. For her whole life a pen had remained a pen. A car had remained a car. Now we were telling her that a line and a circle placed differently were different letters and this did not compute.

If she could walk both directions, why couldn't she read both directions?

Liz's worldview is very different from how I had ever viewed life.

Years later as we remediated ten-year old Liz's reading skills we discovered information from one part of her brain had difficulty connecting to information in another part of her brain. She could spell well during spelling lessons, then ten minutes later the material she knew accurately evaporated and she could not read her spelling word in a sentence. Liz knew she had understood this only moments before and her frustration escalated. Whose wouldn't? Each gift of knowledge felt to her as if it was being stolen from her mind as soon as it was given.

We didn't yet understand generalization and it impact - the need to reteach every lessons in many new environments.

A ROMPER ROOM HOME

During Liz's early childhood we shared our home with a number of infant and toddling foster children. David joined us at eight-months-old. An infant stroke left him paralyzed on one side and social services knew he had been prenatally exposed to alcohol. Because David was unable to use one side of his body we held his good side and encouraged him to utilize his weak side. He cross-pattern crawled to reach Cheerios we placed on stairs and ladders. His favorite daily event and first word was "hot tub." He happily splashed and swam as Karl held his good side. Our knowing David's early brain injury made significant impact in later growth and development.

Indoors we built obstacle courses addressing both children's needs for walking, crawling, jumping and climbing. Sofa cushions, pillows and blankets became mountains and tunnels strewn helter-skelter to encourage exploration. My husband cut peg board into one-foot squares so we could lace them together to make boxes and tunnels. Cupboards were emptied and refilled with pans and bowls. We filled containers with beans, rice and other pouring things for tactile exploration. We brought snow inside in dishpans to build snowmen when it was too cold. We filled sinks with bubbles and water. We washed and re-washed toys in water play. We poured, and dripped, and dropped, and mopped. We spent hours playing with puzzles, and stringing, lacing, and building. We read, played house, danced and sang.

Outdoors we built sandboxes, garden paths, an airplane treehouse and wooden play systems. We stomped in puddles, rolled in leaves, hiked in the magical forest, and enjoyed nature. We swung on the porch swing and lazed in the hammock swing. We dug worms and played in the earth. We watched birds, ants and any other critter that came our way. We bundled up in the red wagon and marched around the neighborhood pulled by our wonder doggies.

Unlike Liz, David thrived on affection and positive touching. He loved being held and cuddled. He and Liz developed a brother and sister bond continuing today. At fifteen months a secure, happy and walking David ran. At seventeen months he had twenty-five clear words and discerned multiple motor sounds. He put the correct pieces into wooden puzzles.

At three, Liz knew sixty breeds of dogs, beat us in putting her puzzles together and loved using "Daddy's big words." She loved listening to stories and playing with David. Then David moved on, as foster children do.

I wainted to go to school.
I thought it would be fun.
I liked Kindergaten. I had
a good teacher.

But in first grade.
I felt dumb. I asked questions
and everyone laughed at me.

I always had to sit by the
teacher. Everyone could read and
I couldn't.

The teacher wrote too
fast on the board and I could
never catch up.

I did not want to be there.

Kid's would tease me and
Say I was the kid with only
10 Spelling words ha ha!

**The clues were there
but we never figured it out.**

**Trouble generalizing behaviors
and information. Verbal language skills
higher than comprehension.**

**Swiss-cheese learning -
Information goes in and slips out.
And so much more.**

I tried the college thing and always failed. I learned it's okay. I am not a highly educated college person. I have to work hard for a little money. Without me people wouldn't look as good. I can't be what I wasn't born to be.

Fran, *FASD Adu*

Liz had great difficulty in:

- *Retrieving previously stored information.*
- *Making associations.*
- *Comparing and contrasting.*
- *Forming generalizations.*
- *Seeing similarities and differences.*
- *Understanding cause and effect.*
- *Walking the walk after talking the talk.*
- *Turning hearing into behavior.*
- *Doing immediately without thinking.*

SCHOOL EXPERIENCES

Liz adapted well socially and enjoyed the crafts, stories and playtime with other children at a small preschool. We enjoyed the respite. Preschool screening determined Liz would benefit from another year at home to catch up on gross motor and auditory processing skills. So Liz remained home and went to preschool the following year while her friends moved on.

We searched for a small kindergarten and found a school of only eighty children in grades K-8. Her teacher was incredible and the children were well-behaved and bright. Liz entered kindergarten at age six, still unable to cut out shapes, hop or skip. While the children practiced memorization, Liz stared out the window. While the children sang, Liz looked at the floor. While the children wrote alphabets, Liz scribbled. But, she excelled at recess. She made friends with her outrageous personality!

First grade was the beginning of a downhill slide. Liz finished kindergarten on a high note. She was excited to attend first grade. We spent the summer playing school and practicing letters and numbers. She boarded the bus the first day feeling secure. She used her 'big Daddy words' during storytime. Then she discovered she couldn't learn to read. Her letters danced on the paper. The other children laughed at her. Her desk was placed next to the teacher to get special help. She began copying other children's papers trying to grasp what was going on. Her teacher grew more and more frustrated. *"Is she lazy? Why can't she learn?"*

Arriving home after school, Liz slammed the door, threw her backpack on the floor and exploded. She quit masquerading as a 'normal' school child. The pressure of the school day released into a snarling, growling, screaming, crying entropic mass on my kitchen floor. I began a daily notebook to document behaviors and statements. We played school before dinner trying to learn what the other children had learned during the day. Our bright-eyed, sparkling daughter who had come so far, now spent storytime curled up in a fetal position. We asked for an assessment, but she was not far enough behind to qualify for special programs. We considered homeschooling and having Liz attend school half days. Her school was very accommodating, but was concerned that her needs were more than they could meet. Liz began to get stomach aches and headaches. School became a nightmare. Her beloved storybooks became her enemies and she no longer wanted us to read to her at bedtime.

My family love just the way I am, but they make me grow, think and do hard things.

They are strict and want to keep me safe. Sometime I get mad about them being strict. Mom and I have secret signals to keep me safe. One signal tells mom I want her to say No. One signal tells me I am out of control and if I want mom to tell me nicely I don't let her signal two times.

if I don't pay attention to her signal she can yell at me.

Parents of children with FASD can help disprove the dysfunctional family theory by attending parent/teacher conferences, becoming active in the child's class, volunteering in the school and attending school activities.

Consistently communicate with the school and your child's teacher.

We decided that public school, with its wide array of services and diversity of teachers was a better option. Liz's new second grade teacher had been a special education teacher in a senior high school and was exceptional. Liz's hand-picked public school third and fourth grade teachers were just as skilled. It wasn't an issue of teacher quality - something was very different and complex with our child.

When other children were learning to read, Liz was struggling with a dancing alphabet. While others were beginning to write stories and short reports, Liz coped with coloring, using a scissor and getting her letters to stay on the line. While others sang *Go You Chicken Fat Go* and exercised, Liz struggled coordinating words with impossible actions. Finally she qualified for an assessment and began Title 1 services for reading and math to help her catch up with other students. Yet even with supports and excellent teachers, information learned yesterday was forgotten today. Her numbers and letters were transposed. The child who worked so hard to love life no longer contributed anything in class, her eyes sullen, her face expressionless.

From her Fourth Grade Report:

"Elizabeth often makes disparaging remarks about herself. She misread words she did know, and then argues about what she had said. Constructive correction is received negatively. In spelling 18 cvc and 2 silent e words, Liz had 25% accuracy. She did not use /th/ or consonant blends correctly. She often used the short vowel and then added another vowel in error. In math Liz was fairly accurate using her fingers for computation in addition and subtraction. She demonstrated knowledge of multiplication and division. In reading she falls below the 16th percentile. Giving her positive comments is very productive. It is also beneficial to let her self-correct rather than marking something wrong."

Liz compared herself to classmates. She thought she was stupid. She hated reading. She hated school. She hated herself. She struggled in group environments. She fell to the floor in rages, used vulgar language and no longer spoke to her family without shouting. Headaches, stomach aches and dizziness occurred daily. She continued to gain weight. She was a very unhappy child. A complete medical exam discovered nothing unusual. Liz, however, compensated for her educational defeats with 'friendships.' Her sense of humor, fascinating playroom and hot tub moved her to celebrity status with her peers and if 'friends' asked her to do something she did it.

I always have lots of friends we liked to have races. I was a fast runner and could win.

I like playing with friends. Our family does fun things, and my friends like being here. We have a hot tub and we had a trampoline. But then mom said too many kids and the trampoline went away.

We also go on bike rides to get ice cream. I like riding bike.

Though outgoing and socially engaging children with FASD are often impulsive, intrusive, overly talkative, hyperactive and starving for attention.

Limited social adaptation is a common problem. Poor judgment leads to exploitation, isolation and establishment of few true friendships, even though they may be surrounded by persons they consider 'friends.'

It is not uncommon for a child to call a list of friends for a play date - and all answer NO!

By the age of nine or ten most children are socialized to cultural norms. Liz was still a toddler on a huge adventure. You never knew what direction she would dash. I felt isolated as I tried to protect Liz from the world and the world from Liz. It was time for a change. Liz would not become handicapped because I was protecting her; she would have to learn to manage in society.

Most children with FASD have trouble taking in verbal instruction, processing the information, remembering what is expected of them and then completing a task. They find it very difficult to master social skills without explicit concrete direction. The next years would mean intense instruction if Liz was to be safe and gain adult interdependence.

By age nine our dreams of academic success for Liz had been crushed. Her bad behavior was escalating and we were concerned institutional placement loomed on the horizon. We didn't have the money to choose to homeschool and yet it seemed to be the only option. The teachers we were working with weren't the problem. They were excellent. I knew Liz was able to learn, but she wasn't learning in a group environment. I kept thinking, if I look back on my life when I am eighty, will it matter more that I built a business or that I raised a child? I restructured my business from over four hundred to ten select clients, left a big office downtown to work at home and study how to teach Liz. We set a homeschool start date eighteen-months away on April Fool's Day, 1997. Liz's job was to try her best during her remaining days in public school. My job was to get my finances in order, keep my select clients happy and learn how Liz learned so I could teach her.

Best friends

Liz explained her school problems: *"Mom, it is like every year the teacher talks faster, and faster, and faster, and faster. I can't hear all the words. I can't remember. I have to make things up. I just answer whatever. I just check off boxes. I don't care if I get the wrong answer. I can't keep up. It makes me crazy. I hate my life."*

Though she was committed to learn to read she placed her real energy into making friends. Once a child who avoided looking at people she now talked to every stranger on the street. Socially we thought we had come a long way. We invited her friends on bike rides for ice cream. We packed picnic lunches for excursions to the park and an older brother purchased a trampoline to increase Liz's gross motor skills, her balance and help her weight issue. Children filled our yard and Liz started a 'friend collection.' Even though she was hard on friendships, children kept coming. She never seemed to run out of young people she considered 'friends.'

Meanwhile, I researched how individuals process information – visual, auditory and kinesthetic. I discovered Liz acquired most of her information through hearing – and her hearing seemed to take in limited amounts of information at a time, miss pieces, and mix things up when outputting that information. I discovered I processed all my information best visually. We were going to be some team – the deaf leading the blind.

Learning To ride a bike was very hard.

I would throw it down and walk away.

When I finally learned to ride I flew over the handle bars when I wasn't looking. I dont know how. and I got hit by a car when a bag got in my wheels and the car didn't Stop. My friend Mikey helped me up.

I didn't See The car. I still don't watch So well. I have a hard time paying attention

It would be years before we would discover that Liz was neurologically living with mixed dominance and what that meant to her abilities, understanding and emotionality.

Meanwhile her feet, hands and mind seemed to be playing a game of charades with her and would get all mixed up. She had difficulty moving in different directions or up and down

Each of us acqu_
slightly different neurod_
velopmental patterns. M_
children and adults who
experience difficulties in
learning, task performan_
or social interaction have
neurodevelopmental
differences which interfer_
with processing. For exam_
ple, when the systems tha_
support vision or the sen_
of position in space, are _
strong enough, then read_
ing, math, general organ_
zation and efficiency may
suffer. Trauma may furth_
complicate matters.

Judith Blueste_
www.handle._

I finally under-
stood mixed dominance
when I stepped off with t_
wrong foot while bowling
and didn't let go of the
ball. I landed face down,
ten feet into the alley, my
ball finally free of my
fingers. I in the gutter.

Jod_

It would be years before I truly learned how to help Liz with balance, coordination and attention issues. My heart broke watching her struggle to be like her friends – to rollerblade, skate, ski, jump on the trampoline and ride a bike. She struggled so hard to overcome her coordination issues and she eventually succeeded keeping hidden for years the hurtful comments she received regarding her clumsiness, inability to skip, her funny hop, run and jumping jacks. Even though hearing was how she learned I didn't know how her auditory processing deficits were affecting many parts of her life. If only I had known then what I know now!

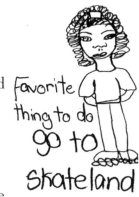

Favorite thing to do go to skateland

While Liz focused on friends and activities. I focused on understanding Gardner's Eight Intelligences and teaching strategies. I wanted to be armed with as many strategies to teach material as possible. I knew Liz could learn, I just had to get the information creatively inside her brain and allow retrievability.

GARDNER'S EIGHT INTELLIGENCES*

Musical/Rhythmic	Rhythm, music, melody. Incorporate music daily, tape record for listening, singing, recording, utilize rhythm and instrumentation.
Mathematical/Logical	Categorize, classify, work on patterns and relationships. Utilize manipulatives, games like checkers and chess, simple machines.
Body/Kinesthetic	Touch, move, interact. Physical challenges, spelling and grammar with dance, math with manipulatives, allow movement and interaction.
Spatial/Visual	Visualize, colors/pictures, map, draw, chart, diagram, puzzles
Linguistic/Verbal	Saying, hearing and seeing words. Listen, appreciate, reading aloud, spelling games, rhymes, tongue twisters, writing.
Natural	Explore, observe, collect, order. Explore outdoors, seek patterns and order within the world, collections, plants, animals
Interpersonal	Share, relate, cooperate, games that problem solve to figure out the knowledge or intent of another, discussion about social interactions.
Intrapersonal	Self-paced, individual, work alone. Express emotions, preferences, strategies, understand wishes, fears and how to cope, cozy quiet spaces.

*Existential intelligence is under consideration

Armed with processing and intelligence knowledge, I still wasn't sure where to begin. Liz had become adept at faking what she didn't know and I was rapidly discovering there were many missing bricks in her education foundation.

I lost my first tooth when I was four. My big teeth came in all over the place. The dentist said I would need surgery and braces. I freaked and cried.

Dental and medical experiences for children with FASD can be very traumatic, not just for the child, but for the parents who are providing support and comfort, and the professionals who are providing care.

Caution must be used in selecting anesthesia, medications and treatments. All medications the child is on must be relayed to the professional; this includes any vitamins or supplements.

Alert professional providers verbally and in writing of any unusual behaviors or reactions the child has previously exhibited. Prepare them, even if they think you are exaggerating.

Roleplay your visit before you go.

Watch your child carefully and document an changes possibly due to medication.

Professionals will need to be able to adapt their methods for the chil sake. While other children began to tolerate being ab to wait for things, handle frustration or deal with disappointments children with FASD continue to struggle regulating their nervous systems as well as their emotions. Huge emo-tional responses can result from discontentment abou anything.

When a change (transition) has occurred, the events of an outing are not within the scope of my son's thinking. He lives in the present. He may however recall them the next day, week, or month.

Viki, FASD mo

ORAL LEARNING

At ages nine and ten, much of Liz's learning continued through oral stimulation. We were constantly dealing with wet sleeves, shirts, chairs, money and whatever else was handy to put into her mouth to help her better understand her world. She still had sucking issues and found her own methods of oral stimulation. She was a chatterbox. Whatever thought popped into her mind flowed out her mouth. Her mouth hadn't had a rest in ten years, except when she was sleeping and even then it sometimes enjoyed a dream-filled conversation. At least we knew what she was thinking.

One day, while I registered for an appointment at the doctor's office, Liz's toddler nose went up in a twitter. She smelled something – most likely the antiseptic smell of a clinical environment. Off she ran, tongue protruding against the clinic's wall, tasting thirty feet of paint and germs. Horrified, I rushed to whisk up the little bundle of energy who now understood why the clinic smelled the way it did.

Another time when Liz was five, the dentist asked her to open her mouth and show him her beautiful teeth. The chocolate-smelling Magic Marker had been well sucked on in the waiting room and a mouthful of brown, discolored teeth glared at him.

As a toddler, Liz was Ms. Biter Extraordinaire. Instead of a kiss I could expect a bite. She would chomp onto my chin and hang on as I pried her off. Our home was filled with apples and carrots we handed to her and said *"people bite food."*

Once Liz picked up Dr. Sagey Puddy Cat the magical 'very much alive' cat, and took a huge chomping bite on his back. Worried for her safety, I picked her up and gave her a swat on the diaper saying *"Do not bite animals."* She had never experienced that reaction and was quite shocked. In perfect FASD style, she turned around and bit me. She did not let go. Realizing this could go on for a long time, I said firmly *"Do not bite people."* I pried her off and put my hands lovingly on her little face looking eye to eye. *"No biting animals. No biting people,"* I reinforced. As soon as I let go she bit herself. Exasperated I said, *"Fine, bite yourself."*

We all learn from our mistakes. First knowledge is vitally important for our neurologically impaired children. What we say is important. I wish someone had told me that all I needed to say was *"People bite food. People eat food. People taste food."*

To this day Liz struggles with biting herself when she is frustrated, scared, angry or in a rage. I wish I could retract those three little words.

MoM asked if there was anything else we could do. The dentist smiled and said, pray. So we prayed for three years.

That dentist died and the new dentist saw all pictures. She was sure to make money on my mouth.

But when I openned my mouth my teeth were perfect. She asked me who fixed your teeth. I told her Jesus. She couldn't believe it.

Dental and medical visits provide two things our children with FASD have great difficulty with: overstimulation and transition

Overstimulation due to the lights, sounds, smells, new people, and necessary procedures.

Transition from the house, to the car, to the waiting room, to the examination room. By exam time we are already down four.

Is it any wonder, they get stuck emotionally and mentally?

We found out eve minor surgeries in the hospital with our son nee anesthesia. The doctors now insist that we stay ir the room wearing surgica clothes. The last time my son fought the 'gas' mask with such force the doctor asked me to coax him and put the mask on him. I succeeded. I also succeede in inhaling enough of the gas so I began to pass out The next time we had a dental check-up, my son had no cavities. I overhea the dentist say, "Thank God!"

Susan, FASD m

Children with FASD seem to be constant ly on the go, never settling down or satisfied. They will move from activity to activity never really focus ing. They may engage in the same type of movemen over and over again.

DENTAL ISSUES

We are attentive to dental hygiene. Our baby's teethe on a soft toothbrush. It's a personal care priority, but tactile defensive children may avoid brushing. We discovered Liz cooperated as long as we did not invade her personal space and made things fun and interesting.

Liz, age one, enjoyed sitting on the bathroom counter, her little feet in the sink, as we brushed our teeth. She chewed a little toothbrush, with her own tiny drop of toothpaste. She watched us make funny faces, laugh and spit in the sink. We rolled our eyes, stuck out our tongues and winked at her. She copied us while standing on the counter, watching herself brush her teeth and make funny faces. We didn't expect perfection, we were attempting to establish lifetime patterns.

Liz, age three joined me on my dental visits. Our dentist let her sit on my lap and watch. He would peek in her mouth as he did my dental work. He praised her as a great dental assistant while she stood on a little stool and held the vacuum to evacuate my saliva. She loved squirting Mom's mouth with the water hose. He let her push the x-ray button. She and the dentist looked at the pictures to decide what to do with Mom. By letting her participate in dentistry, he captured her attention and cooperation. Our normally fearful, rageful child developed a fond relationship with our dentist and he was able to work with her because of this relationship.

Looking back, I should have realized something was unusual when she lost her two front teeth at age four and had the front adult teeth at age five. By age six Liz had most of her permanent teeth and she lost her final baby tooth at eight. Her new teeth were in disarray, jutting here and there within her mouth. Her lower jaw was offset from her upper jaw, her mouth unable to close. Our dentist was very concerned and felt we would need ENT intervention.

Liz went into a FASD dental chair meltdown, as she heard him discuss the orthodontia, tooth pulling and surgery that was to come. I asked if there were any other alternatives. He smiled and laughingly said, *"Well, I guess you can pray."*

Once Liz gets an idea into her head she is immovable. Liz prayed faithfully every night for three years. Today, her teeth are straight and her jaw is aligned, at age nine she had reached her full adult stature. For Liz the sarcastic remark worked. Praise the Lord!

I got a womans body really early too, I was only 8 when I would steel mom's packing tape and wrap my chest so no one would know I wouldn't let any one see me.

The boys would say "did you stuff your bra today" or "you're a big butt!" It was hard to have a 16 year old body and be a little girl.

I just wanted to get out of school so bad and I would beg mom to home school me.

Early adolescence is a difficult time for most youth. Hormones rage as the body changes. Most preteens begin abstract reasoning, enter middle school, seek independence and struggle with identity.

The child with FASD often has a poor sense of self, remains a concrete learner, falls apart with transitions, is impulsive without restraint and makes poor choices of friends and activities. Unless supports are in place teen years are often a time of secondary disability development .

Children with FASD start falling behind more noticeably around the fourth grade. There is an increase in the demands of verbal competence, reliance on reading, and emphasis on abstract thought. The child feels abandoned and isolated. They may become inflexible, rigid and set in their ways. The child often lashes out and attacks the very people who are coming to save them much like a person drowning.

Anger is a normal feeling. It is the choices we sometimes make when we're angry that may not be good. As the parent of a child with FASD, I get angry too. Angry at the overt reactions, at the frustration, at the anger – at the fact that all this was preventable.

Jodee, FASD mom

PRECOCIOUS PUBERTY

Liz began to gain weight and grow after she lost her front teeth at age four. We were encouraged because she had always been very tiny. Looking back, I now understand that the weight gain was the beginning of her changes toward womanhood. If I had only known!

When Liz was seven she informed me she could take care of herself and I no longer needed to help her bathe. She needed her privacy, and her teacher said no one should see her body except the doctor. We told her if she could manage her hygiene we would agree, but if she let herself be dirty or not care for her body, we would intervene. She continued to manage good hygiene and we respected her privacy. Then suddenly our home office packing tape disappeared. Little did we know our eight-year-old was carefully wrapping her chest so no one knew she had breasts and that she stealthfully camouflaged her development with careful hygiene.

Liz reached her adult stature of 5'1" at age nine and experienced first menses at age eight. We thought it was a childhood growth spurt. We never guessed our little girl was stealing her 17 year-old sister's sanitary protection for her own use and that she was too scared to tell us about the sexual statements made by boys who teased and called her names. We had told her she was not allowed to use those words so she did not think she had permission to say them. She continued to gain weight and get more and more sullen and surly.

Homeschooling Liz removed the stress from her life. No longer did she compare herself with other children. I was there to answer questions and provide support. We had hours of one-on-one time, and we focused on remediation, nutrition, health and self-esteem. She loved her trampoline and gained coordination and balance. We jumped through spelling and math drills which helped her maintain focus. Liz was home. Her life finally felt safe, simple and secure. Within the first months of homeschool, she ate well and lost 17 pounds. She was smiling. She was ready for summer. We laughed again.

Precocious or late puberty is common for children with FASD. For the lucky children who develop late, the world allows them more room for their childish behaviors. For children like Liz who was one of the smallest preschool children and a fully developed woman by age nine, the world is not so kind.

When I got angry I used to scratch myself, bite myself, band my head and pull my hair out. Now I know that hurting myself doesn't really help the anger even if it stopped it. I told mom it didn't hurt when I did those things, but the next day it would hurt or I would have black and blue marks.

When I get angry now I go to my mom or pray or bite paper. They help me settle down.

What to do? REMAIN CALM
Keep the person safe.
Limit the number of new situations.
Know your child. Read the danger signals.
Avoid overstimulating activities.
Teach appropriate responses to
overstimulating activities.
Avoid prolonged periods of desk work.
Provide short breaks.
Keep tasks simple, teach with baby steps.
Don't judge the person for a rage.
Love the child unconditionally.
Model mature and safe authority.

"Mom, I have hitters and biters and kickers and screamers inside of me. I need to get them out," Liz screamed. Together we lay on the floor kicking, yelling and banging our fists.

Liz rolled over and hugged me saying, "Mom, we forgot the biters. I think we can save them for another day."

Limbic rage victims frequently kick, spit, gouge, claw, and use obscene language. It is often marked by great strength and speed, making escape difficult. In many, a vestige of self control remains. This may take the form of diverting the rage away from other onto inanimate objects or the self.

Limbic rage is very disruptive to the people who have it and to the people in their environment.

Virginia Scott
The Brain, Fact, Function, Fantasy

BRAIN 'STORMS' - RAGES TO RUN PARENTS RAGGED

For years Liz had incredible rages that lasted from fifteen minutes to two hours. Her body tensed and her face turned fearful as she threw herself on the floor growling, snarling and screaming. A medical exam showed nothing was wrong. We had learned from experience intervention only escalated and prolonged the tirade, so we remained calm and carefully monitored her safety until she got up and walked away as if nothing happened. Public rages were embarrassing as eyes and scowls of judgment scanned our daughter and our parenting ability. Standing in long lines, crowded spaces or unstructured environments like fairs or auditoriums flipped an invisible switch to an electrical 'brainstorm' that quickly escalated. It was frightening and exhausting to watch! Karl and I focused on maintaining our own emotional health — we didn't need to add to her chaos — she needed order to trust control.

I told her that these rages scared me and I didn't know what to do when she had them. I asked her if she had any ideas. Liz explained, *"Mom, I don't know what it is. It's like energy in my toes. Then it goes up my ankles and my legs into the knees. After that I have no control and I can't stop myself."*

"Wow!" I said, *"I think we need a firedrill to stop it as soon as it hits your toes. Let's think of ways to catch this energy."* We decided that she'd say, *"Mom, I need help,"* and I'd put my hands on her shoulders and look her directly in the eyes and say, *"Liz, I love you. You're a really good kid. You are special to God, your family and many others."* She repeated back my statements until she returned words of *"I love me, I am a good kid, or I am okay."* Sometimes I didn't believe her calls for help, or stop to take the time she needed and she'd fall enraged to the floor until her neurological thunderstorm blew over. Then when the sun shone from her eyes and her rainbow smile emerged she'd ask, *"Mom, why didn't you help me?"* My heart broke many times.

Within two months, Liz began talking herself out of the anger before they became infantile rages. Today, she can manage the grizzly bears in her brain when her hormones are balanced, she is rested, not stressed, and is properly fed. We managed Liz's environment as much as possible and watched for the danger signs. Most of all we didn't judge the brainstorms. We loved the child.

Even in adulthood because of her regulatory disorder Liz's anger can quickly escalate. She often acts abruptly or says things she later wishes she could retract. As an interdependent person she continues to work daily on mature responses.

I used lie alot, The words would just fall out of my mouth, then I felt bad and wondered why I said that, I still lie sometimes, but not to my family, Most I lie to be like other kids.

When I was 12 I tried everything, drugs cigarettes, alcohol, Sex and other stuff.

I wanted to be like everyone else. Mom and dad found out and helped me understand why all those.

I believed every one was doing it too.

One day I realized that my child was the cameraman in his life experiences and that was why he never "did" things.

Ann Yurcek - 2007

Two way communication means that both people understand clearly what the other is trying to say. When I speak a foreign language I sound skilled if I am the only one doing the talking, but please don't ask me difficult questions or try to have a conversation.

I wanted to be like everyone else. I wanted people to think I was special too. I am sorry I lie because then I have to pay the consequences. I don't like that

Miko, FASD a

Difficulty with problem solving is one of the reasons persons with FASD lie and steal. They may be sincere in wantin to tell the truth, but not have the faculties availab to relate to others accurately or, in wanting to please, create a fantasy. They know on some leve that stealing is wrong a they will be faced with consequences, but they c not figure out how to bu negotiate or work for it. They behave like a toddl or young child would. Difficulty with communi cation and auditory processing further complica the issue of telling the truth.

THE VALUE OF TRUTH

The virtue of truth is a cornerstone in our foundation. As foster parents, we learned that the children we cared for often had great difficulty with truth telling and so we developed the Truth Counsel table. A Truth Counsel could be called by any family member guilty of any offense as an easy way out of any problem. Truth before being caught by a parent equalled Freedom and Forgiveness. If the guilty person called the counsel and the discussion surrounding the issue was sincere, we granted redemption. If there was an offense done against another, the person presenting the case suggested the restitution to be made and got agreement from person offended.

Once, at age four, Liz announced she was calling a Truth Counsel right this minute! Karl and I took our chairs as Liz crawled up and stood on my chair hiding behind my back. Karl asked her to state her issue. She explained she had toileting problems and messes in her pants.

"Well, what are you going to do about it?" my husband asked.

"I'm going to go to the bathroom right this minute!" she hopped off the chair for the first of bathroom visits every five to fifteen minutes. Our plumbing inspector had emerged to become a nightmare for schools and other programs.

We carefully monitored television, computer and videogames. We drew a hard line between pretend (which Liz doesn't understand very well) and reality. Santa Claus, Tooth Fairy and Easter Bunny were relegated to the same status as an actor playing dress-up. Pretend meant we used our minds for a short time to solve a problem, we didn't use it to fool or trick people. I separate deliberate lying, manipulation or sneakiness – which a person does to remain safe or to hide an action or behavior, and blurting – when words and actions occur as the first thing the person could think of or do. I liken her tales and descriptions to a power surge while I am writing a computer file, the input, never matches the output.

We have been shocked many times with the incredible tall tales flowing fluidly from the mouth of someone who seems to have a limited imagination. We listen carefully to discover what she is trying to say, playing the sleuth by separating and rearranging the patched words to develop the reality. We find her stories mixed with real life or television experiences and her reality of an event seldom matched ours as she can rarely see herself in the picture.

Finally mom let me come home when I was 10 years old.

I learned much easier it was just me and mom. She threw the alphabet out the door, and slammed it shut and we started at the vary beinning, learning in vary little steps. Mom didn't teach me new things until I knew the old things.

I felt safe with mom.

We study all the things other kids study. We go on trips and we cook and make things.

I don't get a frusteated when I learn in tiny steps.

I work primarily with at-risk students. I must rebuild them from the foundations. After six or seven years of failure with our language, they have little or no confidence and less self-esteem. Handwriting is the first area where students believe in themselves again. Success does beget success.

- Jay Patterson

One winter, while turning onto an icy road, I slid across the center lan into bright orange cones. The cones flew helter-skel into the air and Liz exclaimed, "Now, do you know how I feel when I cr my midline!"

I had to laugh.

Liz put forth grea effort to learn and remem ber. Yet, the next day her brain's filing system had the locked drawers and missing files. School was a neverending nightmare.

Inappropriate behaviors interfered with understanding and comple tion of her tasks.

Distractibility, hyperactivity, disruptions and aggressiveness compete for learning time.

Teaching became management task instead a learning opportunity.

SAFE AT HOME BASE

Even with special school services reading continued to pose a major problem for Liz. A friend, who had been homeschooling her child with reading difficulties, told me about *The Writing Road to Reading* by Romalda Spalding. She invited me to attend a week-long training course for teachers scheduled for the summer before I began homeschooling. The teacher, Jay Patterson, consistently achieved two to five year advances in reading with his students and he had stomped through the pitfalls of teaching reading to hundreds of students with difficulties. I signed up hoping to discover ideas to teach Liz.

Jay's adventure began when his nine-year-old son could not spell, even though he read and spoke English fluently. Jay tried to apply his years of classroom experience with his conventional wisdom. It did not work. He searched and found a program that surpassed his expectations. In over ten years, it has not let his students down.

The first day of his training program, Jay shared an essay by Shari Anderson, titled *"Why I Like Spalding Manuscript."* The handwriting was beautiful. The essay, he went on, was written by a student in his English class after two years of rebuilding and reintroducing basic concepts and principles of our language. As he showed the paper a teacher in the front row began crying. Jay knew little about this child's history except that she arrived at his class with little confidence and was plagued by previous academic failure. The school file labeled her MMMI—mild to moderately mentally impaired.

The teacher went on to explain why she was crying. *"Shari was in my fifth grade class. Elementary school was very difficult for her and she chose to do nothing. She would sit and that's about it. She had experienced so much failure in those early years she was afraid of risking success. No confidence. Lots of fear. No desire to risk more hurt. No willingness to try."* The teacher was both incredulous and overjoyed at Shari's progress. She saw this composition as a miracle. My heart soared with hope. Nothing anyone had tried so far worked for Liz in writing, reading or spelling.

Jay Patterson captured my full attention.

"Metalinguistics is a process that transcends the empowering nature of multi-sensory instruction and the four avenues to the brain," Jay began. We needed empowerment. Four avenues to the brain – which one did I miss?

When I get into a problem it is hard for me to get out of the problem. I don't know how I got there and I don't know what to do. Then I freak or yell or say stuff I don't mean. I used to get really angry and lay on the floor and growl. I learned to get angry at the anger getting me.

I also learned that eating good food, sleeping right and vitamins helped turn my special life into good.

As an instructor you keep telling students they are sharp, that their self-discipline and their focusing on details is out of sight. I tell them that they need this precise neurological record to become better readers, writers and spellers. Building dependability, responsibility, and accountability for handling language with care can begin when students are expected to handle something as simple and foundational as the correct formation of letters and letter placement.

Jay Patterson (1999

Every time you se a smidgen of success, you dance in the aisles or on the kitchen table and you celebrate because they have won the biggest game in town. Don't min the neighbors. Just dance.

MOM EVICTS THE ALPHABET

Students learn by what they hear from others, what they see, what they do with their hands and what they personally say from their mouths. These are the four avenues to the brain: visual, auditory, kinesthetic and vocal. I realized Liz learned vocally – the one avenue no one had been letting her use. I immersed myself in Jay's class to learn everything I could. We started at the very beginning.

Dr. Samuel Torrey Orton (1878-1948) a well-known neuropathologist, spent his career researching how the brain best learns language. His passion became researching the reasons why certain students were dyslexic and unable to read or write. From his meticulous studies emerged the well-known Orton-Gillingham and Slingerland programs and the text *The Writing Road to Reading* by Romalda Spalding.

Liz needed to learn her way around a sheet of paper. We began our first lessons in manuscript writing. She learned the page points, short lines, long lines, circles, portions of circles, the clock points and their respective legal definitions. She learned how to hold a pencil, how to sit and how to look at the paper. She learned where to place the paper and keep your head. And then Mom did the unthinkable. In a grand swoop she picked up the dastardly alphabet and threw him out the door. Then she locked it. Liz was hysterical. I had captured her attention and she smiled. I had her curiosity and the beginning of trust, because I understood her pain. We were going to rewire neurons and build her attentional capacity. I had captured her commitment to try. So much for day one. Now homeschool would provide a safe harbor for Liz to repair her broken academic sails.

As we worked with the Spalding method I came to realize that the difference between the names of the alphabet characters and the sounds of their phonemes was too great a leap for Liz. What seemed like simple instruction for others was an insurmountable mountain climb for her. Though she could sing the alphabet song, she was unable to match letters to the multitude of confusing sounds. Liz needed success at handling language at the most elementary level with phonograms (sound pictures), the knowledge that certain letters and combinations of letters make certain sounds in a word. These phonograms became the tiny building blocks to a solid core understanding of reading, writing and spelling. Orton's remarkable neurological research gave us a bridge. Liz had detoured the alphabet attack and come home.

Things were bad for me.
Now I am Tering Not
to do any of them and proud
of it to. I even help the little
kids not get into all that stuff.

Their mom's mom's say
I am an good example. But my
friend tasha's mom says I'm a ho.

Frustration Alert & Stop Program.

1. STEP BACK and STOP !

2. BREATHE. Relax your body and breathe deeply through your nose into your heart and smile "I can".

3. BREAKDOWN the behavior into smaller parts.

   a. **What's my problem?**
   b. **What am I doing?**
   c. **Where am I?**
   d. **Who is affected?**
   e. **How can I change?**

4. Brainstorm ideas to CHANGE.

Discipline is different from punishme because it teaches child to learn from their mist instead of fear and suffe for them. It provides the next step for growth.

I think discipli should be immediate an tied directly and tangib to the reason for the discipline. Discipline th is abstract, deferred, or requires memory, reason, reflection and foresight may not work well.

Bob Schacht, F

Refusing to discipline a child becaus you believe they cannot help their behavior sets them up for failure and you up for unnecessary struggles.

Lori, FASD

I tell Liz chill out! Failure can be an opportunity in disguise.

FROZEN FRUSTRATION BALLS

David rejoined our family as a homeschool exchange student. Diagnosed with FAS he challenged his mother, his school and his family. We'd made progress with Liz in homeschool. Could we also school and care for Dave? No one understands why kids like Dave act the way they do. It is easy to point fingers and assign blame. Dave looks normal and can function normally, at least for a while. FASD behavior is not due to inadequate parenting and many healthy and skilled families care for children with FASD. and the complex behaviors caused by the child's brain injuries and metabolic difference can confound anyone.

One day, reaching my own sensory overload - overwhelmed with not being able to teach, tired of Liz and Dave's self abusing behavior, frustrated with their frustration — I screamed and pulled out my hair. My reaction immediately stopped Dave and Liz and their mouths hung open and their eyes wide. In unison they said *"Mom, are you OK?"* No, I was not OK. I was demonstrating their behavior back to them like a mirror. We spent the rest of the school day setting new strategies.

Dave said, *"Mom, you get mad but you never hurt people. Why did you hurt yourself?"*

And I said, *"Good question, 'why' questions are the hard ones to answer. Let's figure it out."* We came up with things we could do to let our steam out and not hurt ourselves. Asking for help became top priority with praise and prizes for not exploding.

Dave who was eight, made a 'frustration ball' with crumpled paper surrounded by happy yellow tape. He placed it in the freezer to keep it frozen so the frustration couldn't seep out and get him. When he felt frustrated, he took the ball out of the freezer, squished the frustration back into his ball, threw the ball back in the freezer, and slammed the door banning the frustration into a frozen jail.

Liz then eleven, dictated a To Do list to take care of her frustrations: crush cans, crumple paper for the woodstove, take a hot shower, watch myself be mad in the mirror, cuddle in my blanket, close my eyes and breath deeply, jump rope, pull weeds, break sticks for fire, pump the player piano, play with clay, ride bike, go for a walk, dance, count to ten, clean the dog kennel.

We shared these acceptable outlets for the children's frustration with our professional support people, friends and family members. Mom made up her own plan. I gave myself permission to go to my room for time out and Dave and Liz promised to leave me alone for a five minute vacation. *I needed to learn to care for me!*

My mom and sent me to a therapist. She annoyed me and got into my business.

She made me really mad. I hated seeing her. She didn't understand me. She sent me to a psychiatrist who said I have FAS! At first I was mad. Now I know I am not responsible for getting it but I have to learn to live with it.

Nothing was making sense.
Our daughter was an obedient child.
She desired to be good.
She wanted to please.

Yet it felt as though she was
deliberately sabotaging every
effort we made to provide
her love and care.

The fetal alcohol diagnosis made sense.
We <u>finally</u> reached the core issue.
Now that we knew what was wrong,
what could be done?

When we fail to recognize a person with FASD we set up the client and ourselves for weeks, months or years of one frustrating treatment failure after another... When the underlying disability of FASD is recognized, it provides a point of reference for appropriate intervention.

Kenneth Dunning,
FASD dad (1996) FASTime

We struggled with Brain Gym® and cross tapping exercises. Though they helped in small ways we did not see significant improvement until we had results from the neuro-development assessment. When we knew where Liz's development gaps were we began filling missing pieces sequentially. Each step of development needed to be completed to reach the next. Liz needed to learn to cross her midline to be able to cross tap!

THERAPY OPENED DOORS

As soon as we discovered Liz was experimenting with high risk adolescent behaviors, we sought a qualified therapist. We knew we were getting in over our heads – rages, learning disabilities, attachment and adoption issues, anger, resentment, lies, thefts we were managing. But adding sex, cigarettes, alcohol and marijuana all within 17 days of turning twelve we were up to our necks in quicksand!

Therapy provided us a framework to help Liz. Each week her counselor provided homework on a targeted issue. Since it was therapist focused instead of parent focused, the negative emotions were directed at the therapist rather than us. Liz's therapist empowered us to support and encourage Liz as she worked her way through fear, hurt, inadequacy, anger and frustration. We opened doors on adoption issues, peer pressure, and sexuality. We worked as a team to help Liz deal with issues of impulsivity, anger and frustration.

Running late for therapy one day, I dropped Liz off and rushed over to the golden arches to fill her order of two cheeseburgers, fries and a soda. Liz had been calm before I delivered her lunch. She ate it while her therapy session continued and began Liz shouting, jumping, screaming and using four-letter words with the therapist. The therapist contributed no other triggers. Could diet be causing some of our significant behaviors? I made an appointment with a clinical nutritionist and the therapist referred us to a well-respected psychiatrist for an evaluation and diagnosis.

The psychiatrist noted that Liz's history glared with the details of fetal alcohol exposure. FASD had been there all the time, but no one put the pieces together. Her behaviors were symptoms of neurological brain damage. Things began to make sense. I realized professionals only understood separate pieces of our child. Armed with a diagnosis, we sought the best individuals in FASD, traumatic brain injury and learning disabilities. We searched for medical doctors, occupational therapists, physical therapists, teachers, nutritionists and/or neurodevelopmentalist to help us. The diagnosis was a bittersweet gift.

Karl and I alone knew Liz as a whole person – 24/7, 365 days a year and love her unconditionally just because she exists. It would be our job to determine the path to follow in taking counsel from those who had walked this way before us.

But what path? Each person with FASD is affected differently.

We found a doctor who helped me learn how my body works and what to eat to keep me healthy and not have headaches before I would have headaches every day.

Now it happens only sometimes and they are not as bad.

I can't eat wheat or corn syrup or caffeine or MSG at all. At first I thought that was the end of my world.

Now we found other solutions and made up recipes that really taste good. I also lost 37 pounds and I look pretty.

. . . As research unveils the complex biochemistry of the human brain and the intimate connection between what we eat and what we create, this knowledge can enable us to function at our best.

Brain nutrition has four primary aspects each corresponding to a class of food. Like the si of a pyramid, they work together to create, protec power and activate your brain.

1. Structure - Fats for essential fatty acids and cell membrane integrity.
2. Protection - Fruits and vegetables for antioxidants and brain cell longevity.
3. Energy - Carbohydrat for glucose and energy production.
4. Function - Proteins for amino acids and neurotransmitter synthesis.

Basically you ne fatty acids to build your brain, antioxidants to safeguard it, glucose to fuel it, and amino acids interconnect it . . .

MacArthur (199
Nutrition and Your Bra
www.brain.cc

CLEANING THE CUPBOARDS

Liz and I arrived at the clinical nutritionist's office a bit early. Per her usual waiting room behavior, she sat, she stood, she paced, she talked loudly and rudely. Per my usual mothering behavior, I tried to manage her to little avail as we registered, filled out papers, and proceeded to talk with a health coach. The fluorescent lights gave her headaches. She didn't like meeting new people and adding a nutritionist to her repertoire of professionals was offensive.

Our nutritionist, Dr. Brist, had successful experience in working with people with Downs Syndrome, schizophrenia and alcoholism, but had never worked with fetal alcohol exposure. He assessed Liz to determine suspect foods for intolerance and gave us a list of foods to avoid for the next thirty days. My kitchen was going to need an overhaul – wheat, dairy, caffeine, MSG, sugar, preservatives, dyes and corn products were to be eliminated. Liz was overwhelmed and proceeded to hit the walls and melt down in his office. We celebrated the new diet change with our last fastfood sandwich and soda. I returned alone two hours later for a private consultation to learn as much as I could to help my daughter. I promised to find replacements for her favorite foods and over the next thirty days eliminate those suspected of causing her trouble. The doctor committed to research fetal alcohol exposure, nutrition and supplements. We joined forces to see what we could do.

Liz was remarkably less frenetic and impulsive after a month of turning our family diet upside down. Our home was more peaceful than it had been in over twelve years. Her headaches were reduced by half.

Dr. Brist used clear language and remarkable compassion to tell Liz how her body worked and how the nutritional supplements he prescribed could help her body process food and thus help her brain. The psychiatrist assured us we could pull Liz off the supplements and replace them immediately with medication if they did not work.

That first week, Liz exclaimed, "Mom, I can think!" She proceeded to memorize 45 states and capitals, learn her multiplication, understand the concept of division and write a song. Unprecedented!

I like helping my friends when they have problems. When I am sitting with them talking I come up with good ideas and I am really kind and considerate.

I know what it feels like to have problems so I am sensitive to my friends when they hurt. I am a happy person. My eyes sparkle and mom says I shine!

Our children with FASD struggle in a world that doesn't understand their issues caused from central nervous system damage. The very teens who have compassion for a person with visible impairments may avoid or tease teens with FASD because they think they are weird. This is not unusual since teens with FASD are very gullible and naive. They react impulsively without restraint. Authoritative intervention escalates their behavior. As other teens are developing abstract reasoning, our children with FASD remain locked in a child's brain.

She has such a passion for being like everyone else, without a clear understanding of who everyone else is. She chooses inappropriate role models and they become her standard of 'normal.' Keeping her safe is very very difficult.

Knowing Liz ha[s] FASD — neurological br[ain] damage didn't change h[er] behavior, but it did cha[nge] my husband's and my understanding of Liz's world and the frustration she faced in day-to-day living.

We now know:

1. *Memory problems led to her confabulation.*
2. *Frontal lobe problems led to lack of empathy or reading social cues[.]*
3. *Limbic system probler[s] led to blind rages tha[t] surpass logic.*

We provided literature on fetal alcoh[ol] exposure to our family, friends and social group[s]. We talked openly. This [was] not an issue that would disappear.

Liz and I developed a secret FASD signal that alerted her t[o] out-of-line behavior due [to] fetal alcohol exposure.

I believe today, most of what happened to Liz that first week on nutritional supplements, was retrieval of stored information unavailable to her access. In any case, this sudden surge in knowledge gave Liz a new boost of self-esteem.

Liz's stomach aches ceased, her dizziness disappeared, and her headaches lessened to one per week. Her behavior stabilized and we began enjoying Liz's special naive innocence and unusual outlook on life. She started to like herself and try new experiences without her normal negativity. She spoke to us, her eyes sparkled, and her voice was positive. Her weight magically melted off as she ate only those foods her body was able to process well. Teaching her became something I looked forward to. She experimented with new hairstyles and clothes, establishing her own identity.

Liz was able to manage herself within reason. She took ownership of her diet and supplement program. She let me know when she was running low so she did not run out. Her therapist observed her drastic improvement. Our weekly visits became bi-weekly, monthly and then no longer necessary. We had a child we could manage. Could this have happened through diet and supplements alone? If so, did she need all of them? Could we return to some of her favorite foods? I devoured nutritional books. Things were working. I wasn't interested in upsetting the apple cart (the apples seemed to just fall out of Liz's cart all on their own).

I volunteer with youth groups to keep an open perspective on my daughter's strengths, differences and challenges. Working with neurologically undamaged children provides me with the understanding of the areas where Liz needs additional support or remediation. Liz's Cadette Girl Scout Troop headed to the Black Hills, South Dakota for a week of camping – loaded with soft white bread and lots of carbohydrates, incredible environmental changes, daily transitions, and group experiences. On the third day, Liz ran out of one of her five supplements. Fortunately I was there as a troop leader and I assured her it probably would not make a difference. How wrong I was! Within the next twenty-four hours, she attacked me and drew blood, ran away, and reverted to her old behaviors – we had four days to go!

Impulsivity escalated alongside frustration and anger. It became vital that the Troop understand fetal alcohol brain damage, participate in the strategies for her success and provide support to help her regain control. It was the first time I had to expose Liz's neurological damage publically – FASD and its realities.

It was our first beginning step in advocacy.

Now that I am a teenager
I like still being a kid and
sometimes more adult.

I talk with my mom to
learn new things, or when
I am confused or worried.

She listens and help me
understand without saying
big words or a long conversati

She shows me how to do
things different, and we
practice them so I know it
in my heart and my head.

According to Diane Malbin persons working with individuals affected by FASD must try differently not harder

Authoritativeness, aloofness and coldness trigger negative behaviors. My confusion or frustration can magnify my daughter's reactions and place everyone at risk. Every social skill must be taught and retaught. Cause and effect must constantly be reinforced.

Fear can become dangerous.

Impulsivity with out restraint can lead to jail or worse for our chil dren with FASD. The young person often has terrible time comprehend ing the limited freedom given to him by parents. Things can become volat as the child strives for independence and the pa ent adds restrictions. The must be a balance betwee enough protection to be safe and enough freedom to prevent him from dan ger. FASD young people often deny the reality of being unable to make sound judgments.

Barb, FASD m

Growing up, I was always in and out of psychiatric hospitals and was discharged without a clue of what was wrong with me. I would shoplift steal and pull fire alarm. I was easily swayed to do the wrong thing.

Steve, FASD ad

OUR ULTIMATE CONSEQUENCE

FASD does not give a person the license to harm themselves, other people, animals or property. The circumstances of camping bombarding Liz did not excuse violence. My husband and I drew our line in the sand. As an adult she could be jailed and/or fined – her life was already too complicated to include a future criminal record. Society considers her offense assault, her camp behavior qualified as disorderly conduct. We told Liz there would be a Truth Counsel in two days. She was to think about her offense and prepare for a Trial, because 'we the parents' arrested her for physically harming a person. She would appear in front of judge Dad.

During school, I prepared the defendant. We discussed court systems, legal words, and what happens to people who cause harm to others. We discussed what 'under oath' meant and what happens in court if you don't tell the truth.

At our mock trial, Liz presented her case. She was forthright and honest. *"There were extenuating circumstances. I ran out of my nutrients. I was in a strange place. The food was bad for me."* Liz was right she had been dealing with many transitions and changes, however the legal world did not care about the 'how come' just the 'outcome'. Mom presented her side, *"I had asked Liz to get out of the car. She refused. I held her arm. She attacked me, drawing blood. I knew Liz escalates if touched when she is angry, scared or frustrated."*

The Reality: 1. Liz is tactile defensive. Mom knows touching Liz when she is escalating only heightens the experience. Mom knew to back off and return after Liz cooled down. Police would not know that. 2. Liz is responsible for her behavior and not allowed to harm anyone. She will need to learn skills to manage feelings.

The Findings: Liz is guilty of the offense - she must learn not to be dangerous.

The Sentence: Liz is sentenced to house arrest with hard labor, glued to Mom for one month. The sentence can be shortened by one day for each day served with grace. No phone, no friends, no television. All social activities are only with family. Weekend work will be reduced to two hours each day.

Liz got up each morning at 7:30 and worked from 8:00 am to 5:00 pm. She had two 15 minute breaks and one half-hour lunch. She learned many new skills. Of course, this meant Warden Mom was jailed too, but we enjoyed each other and she was free in two weeks. I was her mentor, coach and guide in learning new skills!

My family love just the way I am, but they make me grow, think and do hard things.

They are strict and want to keep me safe. Sometime I get mad about them being strict. Mom and I have secret signals to keep me safe. One signal tells mom I want her to say No. One signal tells me I am out of control and if I want mom to feel me nicely I don't let her signal two times.

if I don't pay attention to her signal she can yell at me.

We have special family signals that help keep our child safe.

One signal tells me no matter what she says she wants my no, to be no, and she is just saving face with her peers.

Another signal says "you are getting out of line, pull yourself together."

PUSHING THE ENVELOPE

Prior to Liz joining our family, I was busy and active, always pushing the envelope. From business success to two hundred mile Canadian wilderness white water canoe trips I had enjoyed the challenges. Now, for over ten years, I had Liz pushing my personal envelope – my patience, knowledge, intuition, human relation skills. She knew all my buttons and discovered some I didn't know existed. Often Liz's needs and behavior push my abilities against a brick wall leaving me with no energy to climb over, dig under or break it down. Family and friends were concerned whether we'd survive parenting this special child. Through these obstacles I came to rely on a personal spiritual relationship with God the Father and His Son Jesus. Many times I was left so empty that all I could do was pray to change me.

I initiated the first Designated Care Giver Law, (revised to the Standby Guardianship Law, 2002, MN Statutes, 257B.01-257B.10) and lobbied it through state legislature. Standby Guardianship (www.standbyguardianship.org) is another alternative for transferring the custody and the care of children to another person. Standby Guardianship allows the custodial parent to make future plans for his or her children without having to legally transfer decision-making power. To date, 22 states and the District of Columbia have enacted standby guardianship provisions in their laws. Though I initiated the law, we had no volunteers to become Standby Guardians for our child. When we asked persons we thought were skilled to provide care, they laughed at us and shook their heads. Their plates were already too full.

I realized I was growing older and at some point Karl and I would face assisted living and independence choices for Liz. I decided to push the envelope back. I set the standard high and held her hand, knowing someday soon I needed to learn to let her go. I immersed Liz in stimulation and experiences becoming her brain coach and life guide. Liz and I stumbled together discussing and processing ways to stand tall. We jumped into society and life with our swamp waders. We maneuvered through laundry, meals, housekeeping, buses and shopping. We tripped over time and appointments, finances and harmful friendships hoping to prepare for the future. I learned to check out an experience or environment before I gave a direction. I learned to teach tiny step by tiny step, stepping back when she didn't need me, stepping forward and catching when she fell. Meanwhile the clock to adulthood kept tick-ticking.

My belief in Jusus, is important to me. when I am alon or confused I can stop and pray and it helps me focus and think of other ideas. I like teen groups and I go to a teen church called the Rock.

The Ten Commandments

SIMPLE MEANING	I LEARN
1. Trust God	Trust
2. Worship only God	To think beyond myself
3. Respect God's name	Power of God's name and words
4. Rest and think about God	To take care of myself & keep myself healthy
5. Respect and love your parents	Obedience
6. Protect human life	To protect life
7. Be true to your future husband or wife	The value of a promise
8. Don't take what belongs to others	Honesty
9. Don't lie about others	Truth
10. Don't want what others have	To be satisfied

For Liz the 10 Commandments are not legalistic or oppressive. They provide her the solid boundaries she needs to live safely.

I'm sure you get judgment everywhere els you don't need it in the church. You made me st and think - am I too quick to judge? We all need to be careful not to judge.
                    Joyce

Liz loves learnir about God, Jesus and H Spirit. She loves the Lor and has her own special relationship. Liz's life is happier when she knows she has votive boundarie that are strong, structur and unbending. A safety fence that provides her freedom with protection. The Ten Commandment written in stone provide that for Liz. A clear a se of rules to measure up to

How do you fin a church body that understands your child has hidden brain dama that causes unusual behaviors? My kid looks so cute!

NO CONDEMNATION IN THE BODY OF CHRIST?

"Why do we kick our wounded?"

After we adopted Liz, we couldn't stay in the church we had been attending. At age two, Liz was very volatile, lost control at inopportune times causing commotion and judgment. Misunderstandings were pervasive. We didn't know what was wrong, so we couldn't help to make it better. Liz wanted to be part of Sunday School like other children. We had to move on.

Happily we found a church where children were mobile as long as they were quiet or participating in the singing, dancing or worship. This church accepted our family as we were and provided Liz the freedom she needed. During the teaching, the children colored pictures or did puzzles. During the worship, the children danced in the aisles, sang the worship songs, and waved colorful bits of cloth. Liz waved and jumped joyfully. I volunteered in the nursery, started toddler Sunday School, and listened to sermon tapes in the car. It was six months before I heard a sermon from the pulpit. Liz had fallen asleep.

One day, at age 13 Liz asked, *"Mom, what is that hot feeling I get right between my lungs when it's something bad."* The Holy Spirit had awakened her conscience. I told her, *"Honey, some people know right and wrong with their heads. You have a special connection with God that will tell you right and wrong inside of your heart. When you feel it, flee and ask God to keep you safe."*

Liz brought her urban friends to our church by the carload. Even within our church's loving framework, they were easily singled out and unfortunately misunderstood and mishandled – their young spirits bruised and crushed. Embarrassed, defeated and hurt, Liz quit bringing her friends and attending church. She decided rollerblading was a better pastime and brought her carload of kids to the rink instead. Thankfully, the church noticed and a teen outreach was started. One hundred and ten teens showed up the first evening. Liz's interest was piqued. "Who brought them," she wondered. She had to check it out. Rollerblades on, in she skated – making a visual 'skatement' – will you accept me as I am? She was embraced back in love. The hearts of the congregation welcomed her, a member of the new generation. I think God laughed. As an adult Liz uses the power of prayer to get through her days, find lost items. settle her emotions and pause long enough to enjoy reflective thought.

My room is my private space. I can let people in but it is mine. No boyz are allowed because mom said NO I like to listen to Mya, Aaliyah, Mariah carey, cash money Records, No limit, Monica, Brittney Spears, destinys child, and much more. I know many songs And like to sing I even sing in front of our whole church.

Personal space and boundaries are important, yet difficult for many neurologically damaged persons to understand.

They may have a limited idea of where their body is in space.

We discovered that the more our daughter is aware of her body, the less intrusive her body placement is to others.

We also discovered how important having her own private space is in order for her respect ours.

FASD is an organic brain disorder. It is not a psychiatric disorder. The central nervous system disorders, growth deficiencies and anti-social behaviors com as part of the package.

How do I keep Liz safe through the teen years so that she enters adulthood with the least amount of secondary disability? How do I teach her the gentle art of living and the dance of life?

Perhaps in time there will be a loving spouse or life coach to walk along side and guide her. Perhaps we will discover new ways to make neural connections and provide her better problem-solving skills, an ability to encode information, and a way t enhance her visual and spatial skills.

Perhaps?

CHOICE AND CONSEQUENCE

Choices and consequences lie at the core of our parenting strategy. Liz was three when David moved on. The car with his new foster mother arrived to take him away. I buckled him into a car seat, hugged and kissed him good-bye and walked in the house. Then as the tears flowed from my eyes, my little Elizabeth softly said, *"Don't cry mommy. He's gone. You know what the problem with babies is? They can't make choices. If he could make choices, he'd still be here."*

Liz has been raised with choices. She also has to live with the aftermath of the consequences of her actions. If she is exposed to limited stress and allowed time to think, she can often make good decisions. The problems arise when she is faced with a new situation, is surrounded by peer pressure, or is stressed. That is not much different from most teens. What is different is her choices are *'off the deep end'* beyond normal comprehension. She doesn't grasp the subtle difference between playing, story making and truth. When friends say everyone is doing it, with childlike naivete, she determines she should immediately partake in the noteworthy adventure. A violent movie or game provides instruction to hurt others and can place a tape recorder of voices and video of pictures in her head. If a friend is across the street and says come on over, she may run across the street without ever looking to see if a car is heading her way. When a light switch doesn't turn on immediately, the switch is destined for annihilation. This impulsivity without restraint is what gets persons with FASD mistakenly labeled behavior disordered instead of regulatory disordered. They get placed into groups that have behavior disordered persons in them with discipline techniques that don't work for neurologically impaired people. People with FASD will stop trying to succeed if they are constantly met with failure and hostility. They may provoke anger and hostility from others, or act out the very hostility they have experienced on innocent persons or animals. It is a vicious downhill spiral – their desire to be kind and good masked with the pain of defeat.

It is vital that we as a society begin to understand fetal alcohol exposure and train individuals who provide education, health care, justice, counseling, and personal care how to care for the individual with FASD. Together we need to discover strategies that work to help persons like Liz make choices to maintain and keep control.

Impulsivity without restraint can become murder.

some of my friends say I act stupid and say really bad things about me.

It makes me feel mad.

Some friends care about me and when I act weird they just say "Ok, Liz you can settle down," or just act weird with me and we laugh and have fun.

We like to go rollerblading at Skateland. I am a really good skater. I like to go fast.

I also like to bikeride and hang out with my friends. We go to the park and swing on swings and talk.

We protect our daughter as much as we can with monitoring and careful supervision.

We strive for open and honest communication.

When she makes a bad choice, we help her deal with the aftermath.

We worry about what will happen in adulthood. Will independence be possible or will it destroy her?

Liz is a kick! Sh loves life and is giving i her all, the way she thir life is. If others don't agree, she just continues her agenda. She doesn't judge others. Things are just the way they are. Li and a lot of other kids have this certain kind of innocence that all of us 'normal' folk could lear from.

Toni Ha

God must be laughing as you are trying to raise Liz. . . .I'll never forget the d she sucked her magnetic nose ring up her nose as we were driving and the resulting explosion. (R) . . .I'll never forget going to the concert and havin Liz hop over the back of the chair and run lost ir the general public. (L) . . . I'll never forget… giggle, giggle, oh my! (K)

Mom's Frie

PEERLESS FAUCETS

We have embraced the teenage metamorphosis of wild hair, creative make-up, clothes, *avant garde* music and adventure. As with each generation, her choices of uniqueness are not her parents.' We realize they are her expression to find herself, and the safest place to find herself is within the love and guidance of a family. Liz will need more time and experience than most adolescents to reach a healthy adulthood. She will fall and fail many times before she reaches a reasonable level of interdependence. It is our job as her parents to love her unconditionally as she faces and meets those challenges – coaching, guiding and walking alongside. We must lift her up as she falls.

As Liz has grown older, friends she held dear have abandoned her. Perhaps fled is a better term. Her unexpected behavior and impulsive statements left them lying in ruins along life's road. Her unusual choices and dangerous actions left them shaking their heads. Neurological brain damage is difficult for parents to comprehend let alone youth. As fast as water can run through a faucet most of her edifying friendships went down the drain.

Liz is an extrovert. She loves life and gives it her all. People are attracted to her, and she easily attracts the wrong people. She doesn't have the discrimination to know the difference. Everyone is a '*friend*,' until she is discarded or betrayed – left with a broken heart. My daughter is resilient. She is a fighter and with the pain of each loss she grows wiser. The experience becomes written upon her heart when it cannot be written in her brain. As her confidant, braincoach and life guide I gently and sometimes forcefully direct her through stormy waters to safety.

Liz deserves what each of us deserves — success, self-confidence, a sense of belonging, self-satisfaction and to be loved. In most cases, this means her environment must be modified to help her function within a safe perimeter as she develops coping skills so she is not trapped by her own behavior.

I gaze down the road five, ten or twenty years, and decide where I hope Liz can be and what things are truly worth fighting for. I have learned I cannot decide what she will do in any given situation, but I can decide what I can do. Unified, my husband and I can decide to choose our battlegrounds in loving, direct and understandable ways for her. There have been many nights over the years we have held each other close as we forge through the mire of FASD.

I didn't think friends would steal from me so told them I had $900. I had saved every penny for five years. my friends snuck in my room and took it. they showed off with it. Mom called the moms and we got some back and the boyz dug a big garden for mom in really hot weather Now I spend all my money. I don't keep any so no one can take it. my friends always beg me for me for money I have worked hard for. I don't want to but sometimes I give them some. they don't give to me money, I don't know why.

Individuals with FASD often don't understand what money means or represents to others. To them taking $100 is the same as taking a penny.

They don't understand the difference between purchasing power and why the rightful owner would be upset if they take it. On the other hand, they are just as likely to give every possession they own away.

My child can be so starved for friends she impulsively calls anyone just to be with someone.

They told me I shouldn't be friends with Liz because she has dumb problems. I told them I have dumb problems too, and we dumb problem people are going to stick together.

I found all the jewelry she had stolen. I was sick. I know I should be prepared for this type of behavior. She has been stealing forever. This tim she could have been arrested. No matter how much we know it is still so hard to accept.

Sharon, FASD mo

What do you mean stranger? He told me his name. He's my friend.

ANYTHING GOES – IN MY POCKET

Individuals with FASD are often five or more years behind in social and emotional development, and model the behavior they see. As a teen, Liz's maturity level was often overestimated and people expected things of her she was not capable of. It has been crucial for us to provide explicit guidance and safe activities by surrounding Liz with positive role models. Liz's real friends tend to be two or more years younger look up to her. Each year, we season our family with an international exchange student. These young people usually provide healthy role models for Liz and give Karl and I a balanced view of mature adolescent behavior.

Liz is not the only child affected by fetal alcohol in our urban neighborhood, she was however the only one diagnosed. We embraced the culture of the neighborhood and befriended the young people. I set my standards high demanding politeness, common courtesy and standard American English. I held each child accountable for his or her behavior. It was not an easy task. I inspected what I expected and they knew it. We found solutions outside the box because there wasn't even a box to look in. Our dining room table was decorated with a baby cactus gardens to eliminate careless stretches across the table. Liz's phone had a timer. More than once I was knighted the meanest mom in the neighborhood. We made it an honor to be part of our family and offered prizes for children with good behavior. Three offenses a child was banned from our yard. We treated the children with respect and trusted with verification. We expected reciprocation. Liz founded the inspirational group the Mo'Angels and for four years I was a roady with a minivan of teens.

It is common for anything not nailed down and some things that were to be found in a pocket. We locked up and hid what we didn't want stolen. I often offered up a simple prayer — *"Lord, whatever is lost, stolen, burned or destroyed, let it be found. Amen."* Remarkably finders always appeared with the missing objects and a smile.

I could not always keep Liz safe and she was the victim of numerous perpetrations since she is easily manipulated by peers. I felt like a mama grizzly bear as I monitored friends, activities and free time. Through tragedies and betrayals she gained wisdom we could not teach her due to results of her poor choicemaking. Yet from these mistakes she has became a thoughtful counselor encouraging younger friends not to make bad choices and defending others being taken advantage of. Through her life challenges Karl and I learned the high cost of innocence and naivete.

I usually hate going on vacations. I don't like leaving my home. I feel safe here.

My family went to Europe and I saw alot of things but it was very hard to be away. Mom and dad bought me a pillow and blanket so I could wrap up and snuggle in the car or air plane.

Mostly we go on motor home trips where I have my own bed.

MoM says we travel so I can learn and understand things better. She says I am a concrete thinker.

We manage the new environment while traveling as best we can.

We find quiet places to unwind.

We pack nutritious snacks and foods she can eat.

We pack books, tapes, games and music she likes.

We pack a surprise bag of fun things. And we stop for bathroom breaks often.

Our kids have amazing ability to bou back from failure, disap pointment and rejectio Sometimes I think thei inability to read social cues, body language, inferences and other non-verbal communica tions is a gift that save their souls and insulate them from a society tha isn't always very tolera and compassionate.

FASlink m

We don't isolat Liz from society we let world experience our wonderful and complex daughter and we let he experience the world.

When people 'really' get to know an understand Liz, they begin to realize normal parenting strategies sim ply won't work for her. Their initial flippant judgment of our inept parenting is washed aw with sincere respect.

GETTING AWAY FROM IT ALL

Once you step onto the FASlane there is no exit ramp and traveling with a young person with a brain disorder does not set the stage for relaxation. It does, however, expose everyone to life beyond the edges of the home turf. Karl and I love adventure. We love the outdoors and the challenges of the sky and the sea. We love the regality of creation.

Liz grew up hiking up and down trails sounding like an Indy 500 race car among the peace and serenity of the wilderness. Homeschooling Liz gave us the freedom to pick up and go when we study a topic to provide hands-on experiences and adventures and we adapted our love of nature and learning to her needs of comfort and security by purchasing an old motorhome. The camper provided us the safety and comforts of home, with the flexibility and independence to explore. Whenever Liz was overstimulated, we returned to our home on wheels. By traveling in the motorhome, we were able to visit battlefields, explore beaches, caverns and waterfalls. We enriched our lives with history in living museums, geography on the road and nature in state and national parks.

Faced with a school district curriculum guide to teach Viking, Roman and European history, we decided to visit our previous foreign exchange students to create a backdrop for understanding. We stretched twelve-year-old Liz visiting Iceland, Denmark, Sweden and Germany. We walked in Viking and Roman ruins, explored monasteries and castles, wandered through orchards and climbed mountains. Liz was surrounded and struggled with lifestyle and language differences and her behavior reverted to survival. Around her neck hung her house key and a pacifier. Her main focus – is there food, is there a bathroom and where will I sleep? We worked hard to maintain her rest since transition and change are extremely difficult. Our first purchase was a down comforter and pillow with sheets to match her bedroom. From the first day she knew she was returning home and like a small child she cocooned herself into the blanket. We carried food and water and our first tourist stop was always the toilet. Once Karl performed superhuman heroics as he swooped her off the departing train. Her impulsivity and impatience led her to jump alone onto a Stockholm subway heading the wrong way. She was right next to us!

Hands-on experience proved to bridge Liz's understanding of her world and enabled me to teach her while we got away, but not off – the FASlane.

Everbody love camping trips but I hate it. it's cloud, it's uncomfortable the tents stink, the food makes me sick and everything is different than home. I do not like overnights ffor Scouts or church

We went to the Bahamas. I like it because it was nice weather there were big beaches and the people were really nice to me. We had our own condo so I had my own space. and mom could cook food I can eat.

Choosing to embrace the wonders of the world with a child who has hidden neurological damage exposes a family to unwarranted public misunderstandings of inappropriate parenting or discipline techniques.

Our special high risk children do not need their lives further complicated by an unnecessary intervention or removal from our homes by child protection. It is prudent to develop a small parenting manual with approved and written strategies from professionals that you can share with other care givers.

We discovered w. we did the evals with To. Hager that Liz had mixe. dominance issues:

1. *Visual processing difficulties affect the awareness of what is going on around her and the ability to interact socially.*

2. *Auditory inefficiencie. make it difficult to follow directions, pay attention to what is said, and interact socially.*

3. *Behavior that is a reflection of auditory processing hinders her ability to make sense of her environment, ta. appropriate actions and achieve academic. In addition, she is ofte. disconnected from her feelings and unable to. express reasons for out. bursts or misbehavior.*

And these could be remediated with the right therapies?

Liz is an experienced primitive camper and has survived numerous Boundary Waters Canoe treks. Church camp and Girl Scout camping were a whole different story – twenty girls, imperfect showers. Liz often provides her own solutions to cope with environmental elements that present challenges. It didn't surprise me she claimed my car as her tent and chose not to climb to the mountain peak. In doing so, she kept herself and the other girls safe from her impulsive behaviors. There is usually logic in Liz's choices, though it may be a challenge to find or comprehend it until I step back to silence by unfiltered defenses and frustration.

We discovered a condo unit or the camper provided the same sense of security for Liz we had at home. We stayed in one place. We shopped for food. She ate without the overstimulation of a restaurant. She had her own bed. We maintained our family structure and schedule. In a condo community we alerted neighbors of our daughter's issues and they became friendly supporters for a successful vacation.

Traveling with Liz is always an adventure. She has no internal clock. Time is abstract to her and she does not comprehend how it works. If we are to be somewhere at a certain time, she is just as likely to think she should begin getting ready as she is to be ready. We are often late. Fortunately, she lives in a family who manages well on process time versus clock time. On the last day of vacation her internal clock says "we are going home" and the day starts when she wakes up. Unfortunately, she is likely to wake to go to the bathroom at 1:26 am. It is the new day and time for 'everyone' to get up. So much for sleep.

Airplane travel is filled with intense sounds, smells and feelings. A person with tactile defense issues may have difficulty with the limited space, turbulence and pressure changes. Once Liz's ears filled with pressure on landing. She was drinking spring water and took the bottle and poured the water into her ear. Then she shook her head and hit her head on the seat. At that point the fumes of verbal four letter exhaust spewed from her mouth and she threw the bottle – still filled with water – into the air. It was now raining in the airplane. The seat next to me was drenched.

As if nothing had happened, she shook her head and smiled, *"Whew, that's better! I'm going to do that on every flight."*

It is difficult to access each new situation and discover how it can become a 'teachable moment' for a safe and positive growing experience. Let me dry off first.

When I was little, I wanted to play harp. I still play but I had a real hard time.

Mom wouldn't let me quit. She says it helps my math. She says I need to learn I can't quit hard things. I think life is hard, but I can't quit.

Mom says I am important and God has a plan for my life.

Special Features of the Suzuki Method

Parent involvement
Listening
Repetition
Encouragement
Learning with other children
Early beginnings
Graded repertoire

Much of what I learned in teaching Suzuki I carried over to other subjects. The most important lesson was . . . tiny step by tiny step !

Dr. Suzuki developed his method to help children fulfill their capabilities as human beings, not to produce professional musicians.

Playing an instrument does not come easily for Liz. We teach her only three to four notes and one tiny new thing at a time. The Suzuki method breaks each song into hundreds of learning opportunities so we can focus on many different things within pieces she already knows. We provide rewards for a positive attitude, practicing and attending musical events.

Liz enjoyed group lessons until she discovered that children who began harp instruction two years after her, had moved beyond her skills.

SUZUKI — THE ART OF LISTENING

Liz loves music. As a small child she laid on the couch and told us her ears were "eating the music and putting it into her tummy." Liz's older cousin plays beautiful harp music and inspired Liz to to play the harp. We decided to introduce Liz to harp music instruction with the Suzuki method.

Dr. Suzuki believed musical ability is not an inborn talent, but a talent that can be developed. Any child properly trained can develop musical ability in the same way most children learn to speak their mother tongue. The potential of every child is unlimited and in teaching the child music, we are creating a medium for emotional and spiritual growth. As he said, *"Teaching music is not my main purpose. I want to make good citizens, noble human beings. If a child hears fine music from birth, and learns to play it himself, he develops sensitivity, discipline and endurance. He gets a beautiful heart."*

The ideas of parental responsibility, encouragement, listening, and constant repetition are some of the special features of the Suzuki method. The parents become the 'home teachers' and learn to play and teach the child. The child's efforts to learn are met with sincere encouragement. Each child learns at a individual rate, building on small steps to master each step. There is no set time plan to the learning. The general atmosphere is enjoyment, generosity and cooperation. Steps are repeated continuously throughout the program to provide reinforcement. Each child plays the same repertoire of music encouraging younger children to play what older children are playing. In addition, Suzuki students develop basic competence on their instruments before they read music.

Children as young as three or four-years-old learn to play an instrument by ear using the Suzuki program. Liz was already seven, far older than most of the beginners and struggled with auditory processing deficits. We wrote to MacPhail School of the Arts in Minneapolis and provided details about Liz and her desire to play. They blessed our family with an instructor who was the first chair harpist from the Minnesota Orchestra willing to do private instruction in her home to decrease stimulation. The skill of teaching three and four-year-olds blended well with finding ways to creatively teach Liz. The hard work of learning music strengthened the paths between the right and left hemispheres of her brain and improved listening skills.

Today, Liz has a fine ear for music. She spent six years in Book One.

It is hard to learn new things with out getting frustrated.

I don't like school even if I am homeschool with my mom. I hate math and feel stupid at it. I have to work too hard. I don't like why questions and Science is the worst.

I know mom tries to make it fun but it is not.

The central nervous system has four main functions:

1. To RECEIVE information through the three main sensory channels of tactile, visual and auditory.

2. To PROCESS (understand, interpret or categorize) this information through auditory and visual short-term memory.

3. To STORE into the long-term memory.

4. To UTILIZE the input.

Connections must be available !

Neurodevelopmen philosophy implies a continuum of function ranging from a low of coma to a high of genius All children are on this continuum.

It further believes that:

1. Function provides a mirror from which the level of development may be evaluated.

2. Development of the system follows an orderly sequence.

3. Everyone moves through the same development steps only at a different rate; some skip steps which can cause inefficiencies

4. The most credible experts of any child are their parents.

Robert Doman,
www.nacd.o

PLATEAUS AND HORIZONTAL LEARNING

I structured Liz's schooling for success, but by age 13, it appeared we'd hit the vertical peak the psychiatrist warned me. Did I need to figure out horizontal learning strategies? Was there a way to press on? I discovered Toni Hager on the Internet. Toni studied under Robert Doman, Jr., who worked in the development of over 15,000 home based neuro programs for children. She worked with the neural plasticity of the brain - rebuilding neural highways. She believed that *"Academics are developmental levels. You are capable of teaching your child the academics of writing, reading and math, when the brain is at that level. If the brain hasn't reached a certain developmental level, it will not learn academics at that level."*

What level of development was Liz's brain? Could Toni tell me? I called her. Toni was traveling through Minneapolis with a one hour layover at the terminal. I sent her Liz's manuscript for this book. She sent me all her articles. She laughingly told me when we met *"Liz is the first client I've had who gave me a detailed written history on her own. From what I already know about her, I have some things I can show you today. I brought you the 'Brain Builder' computer program and some training tapes so you can begin working with her immediately. I will be back through town in about a week. Why don't you bring Liz so we can meet."*

Neurodevelopment is based on the developmental profile. The profile represents functions associated with parts of the central nervous system. When the brain is given enough input, then it provides appropriate output. In order to help Liz, we needed to discover where the gaps in her development were. Toni did a functional neurological evaluation analyzing mastered skills and functions at each development level. She carefully noted which functions were absent or inefficiently performed to chart what part of the central nervous system was dysorganized. From this information she began to design Liz's program. *"There is no guarantee we can do anything."*

Toni taught me on the first day basic exercises to begin to build a neural highway back to Liz's brain. They were easy to do, didn't take a lot of time and Liz liked them. Liz and I began the new exercises and started working on Brain Builder, which we nicknamed Brain Buster. Her initial auditory and visual digit span began at 3-4. Liz had been processing her information at the level of a three to four-year-old. If only this could help her! Had our Creator made a blueprint we could build from?

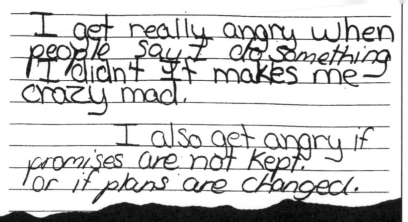

I get really angry when people say I do something I didn't. It makes me crazy mad.

I also get angry if promises are not kept, or if plans are changed.

In order for the brain to process information it must first have the ability to hold individual pieces of information together – short term memory.

The 'normal' two-year-old understands only two-step directions (get shoes, eat dinner, go ride) and speaks in couplets (want eat, no bed). A three-year-old processes three (simple phrases); a four-year-old, four, and on up to a seven-year-old to adults. A seven-year-old or older should be able to understand seven bits of information. That's one reason phone numbers are seven digits.

The individual above age seven who holds 3, 4 or 5 pieces of information together is struggling - to learn, to behave, to function in normal life

Everything affec the brain to some degree The brain's physical environment, general health, allergies, sensitiv nutrition and respiration play an enormous role in the brain's ability to receive, process, store and use information. The rea tragedy is that individue are attempting to cope with unidentified neurol ical dysorganization tha does not need to exist.

Behavior is a reflection of auditory processing. Behavior is th ability to make sense fro the environment, make decisions, take appropria actions and achieve aca- demically. A ten-year-old or adult who can process only 4 or 5 pieces of infe mation will whine and throw a temper tantrum like a four or five-year-c when he or she is stressed overwhelmed or being to "No".

Infants develop from head to toe, shoulders to fingertips, hips to toes and internal to external. Neurodevelopment looks at how the brain receives, processes, stores and utilizes information. Output is a reflection of input. The evaluation included the receptive areas of visual, auditory, and tactile channels including processing; as well as the expressive areas of manual (arms, hands, and fingers), mobility (legs and feet) and language. The evaluation also included social/behavior competence and nutrition. Academics were assessed one-on-one with national testing standards. Liz (age 13) thought the evals were fun. What we discovered was eye-popping.

Liz, who was a failure-to-thrive infant, had never learned to roll over or cross crawl, but she walked. No wonder coordination was an issue. She could not hop, skip or do jumping jacks, but she ran and jumped on everything. Toni gave us exercises explaining that these skills also affected other development and life skills. Within two weeks Liz could cross pattern crawl, hop on one foot with her eyes closed and easily roll over. Her reading began to flow and she requested opportunities to read.

Liz's pupils did not constrict or dilate when exposed to light. Toni gave us exercises to help her pupils begin to open and close. At first, she had trouble opening her eyes for the exercises. Within a week she was less sun sensitive and able to use a computer without getting headaches. She could begin to learn to type.

Liz lacked tactile sensitivity. Toni taught us to utilize all the tactile senses - light touch, pressure, pain, friction, hot and cold. Within five weeks I was writing word messages on Liz's back with a feather. She was receptive to tickling. She had never had reflexes in her legs and they were jumping. She **asked** me for a hug!

Liz had learned work-arounds in areas of basic academic skills. Toni found the gaps I didn't know were there and taught us to fill them. Liz began developing automaticity in areas of word recognition and mathematics.

A child's brain needs 50% of the oxygen it takes in. Liz was a mouth breather and her brain needed oxygen. She began to learn to breathe through her nose. At first she was afraid she die of suffocation. She lived, and walked, and soon sprinted while nose breathing.

Thirty-one neurodevelopment exercises later, Toni said *"Well, that's enough for this time. Let's see what Liz can do with these."* At eight weeks into the program, Liz's digit span was a solid 5-6, a jump of two full development years. We were not on a plateau. We were at the base of the mountain ready to climb with a new trail map.

I am really good with hair. The people at the hair store call me Sparkles and like my ideas. I like to buy hair pieces and weave.

When I want to work with hair or be a singer or be an actress, or clothes designer.

I know it will take a lot of work to do that. I probably can not be everything but I can be the best I can be.

*Many find a solution to life's problems in a drink of alcohol. As you can see the result is far from easy. We need to face the fact that alcohol **does** damage a child's brain.*

Liz is a gift not just to our family but to the world. She has enriched my husband's and my life. She has stretched our minds, our personalities and our hearts. She has challenged us to be better than we ever had to be.

A Place in My Mind

Once upon a time
    The sky was so bright
    in a place in my mind.
Days have passed
    and sorrow has come.
I'd like to take
    that time today, but
    time has passed away.
Dreams have died
    like someday you and I
In my mind is like a drea
    just showing you how
    much you mean to me.
I know your face will
    never show a smug or
    tear deep inside
    how much you fear.
Your smile is like
    a rainbow
    with many colors.
I just want you
    to know
    I love you so.

Liz Ku

1/24/2000 her first po

"Mom! I got a seven
Brain Builde

3/2/20
seven weeks on progr

MOUNTAINS TO CLIMB

Our family has grown together on this FAScinating journey. Karl and I have learned to live, feel and understand Liz's world. We have set attainable standards and modified our environment to meet challenges head on with success. We are not always successful. The trials and struggles of parenting a child with FASD can be overwhelming. I am grateful to have a life partner to walk this path with me because I don't have the strength to do it alone. I give each day to my Heavenly Father, it's successes and it's problems. I Glorify God in the dark time and I ask for His wisdom, protection and peace. I am eternally grateful for His guidance.

Liz has been surrounded by support services and unconditional love. We hope a life coach or a spouse will eventually take the baton we hand over. Neuro-research is receiving better funding and discoveries are being made daily. The internet has connected researchers, medical professionals, scientists, nutritionists, alternative health practitioners, neurodevelopmentalists, parents, therapists and educators.

Trailblazers have gone before us – doctors, scientists, researchers, teachers, judges, advocates, writers, therapists. We, with our children, are the pioneers – planting and harvesting new ground in the fields of prenatal alcohol exposure. This is only an epoch. We have crossed the prairies. The mountains lie ahead to climb and move. It will be our children who move them.

New Year's 2000, Liz asked me, *"Mom, what is your goal for the next ten years?"*
"My goal for the next ten years is that 65% of young people with FASD have successful lives instead of 10% like today." I answered.
"Mom, my goal is 90%. Sometimes I get mixed up and confused. I always try to be a kind and good person. When I get married, I want my husband to know everything about me and FASD so he can be supportive and understanding and not get frustrated by my behavior. Like when I act weird or lose control. Or when I feel horrible because I blow it or can't understand. I guess my boss will need to know about it, too. Because I get confused or frustrated. FASD is not going to stop me from living the best that I can. I love you, Mom."

I love you too, Liz. You will be your best, I know you will.   Mom

FASD RESOURCES FOR FAMILIES

BOOKS

For Medical Professionals

Brick, John, Ph.D. *Handbook of the Medical Consequences of Alcohol and Drug Abuse* (2004) The Haworth Press

Golden, Janet, *Message in a Bottle - The Making of Fetal Alcohol Syndrome* (2006) Harvard University Press

CDC - Center for Disease Control - Download Fetal Alcohol Syndrome Guidelines for Referral and Diagnosis http://www.cdc.gov/ncbddd/fas/documents/FAS_guidelines_accessible.pdf

BRAIN books you can understand

Amen, Daniel G. M.D., *Change Your Brain, Change Your Life, The Breakthrough Program for Conquering Anxiety, Depression, Obsession, Anger and Impulsiveness.* (1998) Three Rivers Press, New York, NY

Diamond, Marian, PhD., *Magic Trees of the Mind: How to Nurture Your Child's Intelligence, Creativity and Health Emotions from Birth Through Adolescence* (1999) Plume

Doman, Glenn J., *What to Do About Your Brain Injured Child?,* (1994) Paragon Press, Honesdale, PA

Elliot, Lise, Ph.D., *What's Going On in There? How the Bran and Mind Develop in the First Five Years of Life.* (1991) Bantam

Goldberg, Stephen MD, *Clinical Neuroanatomy Made Ridiculously Simple,* (1997) MedMaster, Inc., PO Box 640028, Miami, FL 33164.

Thomas, Dr. René ,D.C.,N.D., *Powerful Food for Powerful Minds and Bodies A Family Handbook on Nutrition* (2004) Hampton University Press

Lyon, Michael R. MD, *Healing the Hyperactive Brain Through the Science of New Functional Medicine* (2000) Focused Publishing

O'Brien, Dominic, *Learn to Remember, Transform Your Memory Skills* (2001) Six time World Memory Champion, Duncan Baird Publishers, London

Robbins, Jim: *A Symphony in the Brain, The Evolution of the New Brain Wave Biofeedback* (2000) Atlantic Monthly Press.

Scott, Susan: *The Brain: Fact, Function and Fantasy.* (1997) (Must be ordered from the author) Northwest Neurodevelopment Training Center, Inc., PO Box 406, 152 Arthur Street, Woodburn, Oregon, 97071. (503) 981-0635

Sacks, Oliver: *The man who mistook his wife for a hat and other clinical tales*, Summit Books, NY (1985) *An anthropologist on Mars; Seven paradoxical tales*; Alfred A. Knopf, NY (1995)

Stine, Jean Marie. *Double Your Brain Power. (*1997) Prentice Hall Press.

EDUCATION help children learn

Blow, Susan E., Elliot, Henrietta R. *The Mottoes and Commentaries of Friedrich Froebel's Mother Play.* (1895) D. Appleton and Company. New York

Campbell, Don G. & Brewer, Chris. *Rhythms of Learning Creative Tools for Developing Lifelong Skills.* (1991). Zephyr Press

Greenspan, Stanley I M.D. & Wieder, Serena PhD: *The Child with Special Needs Encouraging Intellectual and Emotional Growth.* (1998) Perseus Books.

Greenspan, Stanley I M.D. with Breslau, Nancy Lewis: *Building Healthy Minds, The Six Experiences that Create Intelligence and Emotional Growth in Babies and Young Children* (1999) Perseus Books.

Kline, Peter. *The Everyday Genius, Restoring Children's Natural Joy of Learning – And Yours* Too. (1988) Great Ocean Publishers, 1823 North Lincoln Street, Arlington, VA 22207.

Pierangelo, Roger, PhD. 1996. *Parents' Complete Special Education Guide. Tips, Techniques and Materials for Helping Your Child Succeed in School and Life.* The Center for Applied Research in Education.

Tobias, Cynthia Ulrich. *Every Child Can Succeed.* (1996) *The Way They Learn* (1994) Focus on the Family Publishing

Shapiro, Lawrence E., PhD: *How to Raise a Child with High EQ, A Parents Guide to Emotional Intelligence.* (1998) Harper Perennial.

FASD RESOURCES FOR FAMILIES

SUPPORT AND INFORMATION

NATIONAL FAS DIRECTORY www.nofas.org

International Fetal Alcohol Awareness Day
"Ring Those Bells" September 9 @ 9:09 am – www.fasworld.com

ARC – FAS Resource and Materials Guide. http://thearc.org

Alaska Program on Fetal Alcohol Syndrome www.hss.state.ak.us/fas/

ARBI – Alcohol Related Brain Injury FASD Resource Site www.arbi.org

Better Endings New Beginnings www.betterendings.org

CDC – National Center for Disease Control www.cdc.gov/ncbddd/fas/

FASALASKA www.fasalaska.com

Fetal Alcohol and Drug Unit - WA www.depts.washington.edu/fadu

Fetal Alcohol Syndrome Diagnostic and Prevention Network - WA www.depts.washington.edu/fasdpn

Fetal Alcohol Syndrome Community Resource Center www.fasstar.com

FASCETS Fetal Alcohol Syndrome Consultation, Education and Training Services www.fascets.org

FASlink helps families dealing with fetal alcohol. Great downloads. www.acbr.com/fas/

FASFRI – Fetal Alcohol Syndrome Family Resource Institute www.fetalalcoholsyndrome.org

FEN – Family Empowerment Network: Support for Families Affected by FAS/FAE

MOFAS – Minnesota Organization on Fetal Alcohol Syndrome, (612) 803-8746. www.mofas.org

NOFAS – National Organization on Fetal Alcohol Syndrome, (800) 66-NOFAS. www.nofas.org

NIAAA – National Institute on Alcohol Abuse and Alcoholism www.niaaa.nih.gov

SAMSHA – US Dept. Health and Human Services fascenter.samhsa.gov/ 1-800-662-HELP (4357)

This list is provided to give you a connection to links, support, education and information on fetal alcohol. It is by no means conclusive, nor does the author endorse everything these sites represent.

ON-LINE FASD SUPPORT GROUPS

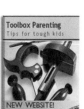

www.fasstar.com Teresa Kellerman offers sound advice and support connections

www.fasflight.com Run by Stephen Neafcy an adult with FASD advice and support connections

www.toolboxparent.com Collaborative site run by Deb and Nate Fjeld and Jodee Kulp

PARENT/TEACHER STRATEGIES

www.difficultchild.com The Nurtured Heart Approach by Howard Glasser author of *Transforming the Difficult Child.*

www.disabilityisnatural.com Kathie Snow provides professionals and parents with a wholistic and healthy viewpoint of raising a child with a disability.

www.tagteach.org Karen Pryor offers an innovative idea for top athletes and students.

www.knarlwoods.com Jodee and Karl Kulp's Knine&humanKIND Brain Booster Buddies.

FASD RESOURCES FOR FAMILIES
KULP TREASURY

As parents we pledge to:

- Strive to keep our young people safe.
- Focus on positives rather than negatives.
- Respect individuality in each person.
- Allow freedoms as responsibility, judgment, new skills and talents develop.
- Show we value each person's work and provide opportunity for learning.
- Not criticize or squelch a person's enthusiasm though we may need to redirect it.
- Help each other deal with failure and bounce back without being devastated.
- Talk about a person's strengths and figure out ways to maximize them.
- Provide support systems.
- Provide logical consequences.
- Keep ourselves healthy so we can be better parents.
- Accept FASD is going to change our life in ways we cannot control.

We make the commitment to each youth in our care that if they find themselves in trouble, they can call us and we will come and get them…no questions asked.
We discovered long ago they are so glad to see us, we usually get details before we get home.

We determine family signals that keep everyone safe and respectful.
For some of our kids these have been very overt, and for others very subtle.

The table is safe for any discussion. If you bring an issue to the table before we catch you it will be discussed amicably.
This has always promoted honesty and openness in our family.

We strive to find the 'right' balance of freedom and discipline for each family member.
Each child is on a different time line for being able to do things, and each child requires different discipline.

Tips:

- Discover your child's personality, learning and processing preferences.
- Don't discount the impossible. Children can surprise us. Things that irritate you now may lead to a future success for your child.
- Provide exposure and experiences. Coach and mentor them through life's challenges.
- Teach them slowly. Teach them patiently. Teach them again and again. Do not sacrifice the quality of your teaching to encourage quantity. (When I teach Liz housekeeping skills, I study how professionals clean and teach her professional methods.)

FASD RESOURCES FOR FAMILIES

TREASURE HUNTERS

My child hates herself, thinks she is stupid and ugly...

what can I do?

My heart breaks for the self-esteem of these children. They try so hard to cloak themselves in a mask of normalcy and then dive into a social abyss with their dismal behaviors. They are misunderstood, misdiagnosed and struggle with normal daily life issues.

We went on a treasure hunt for both Liz and David. We wrote a proclamation and presented medals to each child. We posted our results on the refrigerator. We gave a copy to David's mom, to Liz's therapist and we told Grandma and Grandpa! We held parties for success!

You won't regret going on a treasure hunt for your child.

Common Good Qualities has been compiled from ARC Northland in Duluth. Their sources were from Clarren, Streissguth, Morse, Malbin, Rathburn, FAS Resource Coalition.

Common Good Qualities and Talents of Persons with FASD.

tactile and cuddly	friendly/happy
spontaneous	loyal
trusting and loving	gentle
affectionate	curious
persistent	willing
involved	loving of animals
enjoy gardening	enjoy constructing
kind and caring	helpful
concerned	sensitive
athletic	moral and fair
artistic	musical
highly verbal	rich fantasy life
hard workers	atypical strengths
nurturing	compassionate
sense of humor	committed
devoted as parents	determined
strong sense of self	creative
social	follows through

good with younger children

wonderful story tellers

good long term visual memory

Tips:

- What turns your child on? What are the child's keen interests or talents? Does your child know something no one else in the family does? Let the child teach others.

- Does the irritating behavior demonstrate creative problem solving? Salesmanship? Leadership?

- Try to provide ten positive comments to every negative comment you give your child.

- If the child is having trouble learning or understanding something, take a deep silent breath, break it into smaller pieces and when they conquer the first piece rejoice and go on to the next.

- Don't hinder the caterpillar from growing into a beautiful butterfly.

FASD RESOURCES FOR FAMILIES

TEACHING TIPS

1. Observe, refocus, reframe.

Misbehavior is often a neurological misfire. Take a deep breath, think about what might be going on. Is it the child can't or is it the child won't? Ask the child how you can help. You may be surprised at her answer.

2. Give your child only one direction at a time.

Multiple directions are confusing to a child with FASD. The student may forget what was said first, may not understand what was said or may be confused by a two or more part question. Keep it slow, keep it simple.

 a. Give clear directions - say "put your coats on" instead of "get ready to go."

 b. Use fewer words - stop, walk, go.

 c. Have child repeat back what you say.

3. Model and mentor correct behavior.

Focus on behaviors you want the student to grow, not on behaviors you don't like.

4. Reteach, reteach, reteach . . .

Keep it simple....if they are not getting it break it down into even smaller pieces or teach something easier to build upon.

 a. Use repetition.

 b. Be consistent.

 c. Make smaller steps.

 d. Build on learning.

 e. Try backward chaining.

5. Teach replacement behavior.

 – Reframe

 – Thought-stopping, positive thinking

 – Deep breathing and relaxation

 – Fun, humor and laughter!

6. Use Motivators.

Encouragement, positive attention, rewards and incentives for appropriate behavior and meeting learning challenges. Set a goal to be accomplished. Some incentives work well small toys, money, time with friends, roller rink passes, special dinners, and movies.

7. Modify your environment for the child's success.

Discipline yourself to be sensitive to set up your child for success. This may mean changing plans if the child is too tired, irritable, or nervous. Never go out hungry or over stimulated. The environment is an absolute 'key' to the child's success. Prevent the meltdown from happening.

8. Keep yourself healthy.

Maintain the support of other teachers. Teaching children with FASD can be very frustrating.

9. Be a team player.

The parents of a child with FASD will have ideas of how to help you with their child. Listen carefully to what they have to say. Find a way to keep in touch with the family on a regular basis.

10. Laugh and have fun together!

FASD RESOURCES FOR FAMILIES

TEACHING RESOURCES WE HAVE USED

Can Learn
www.kidscanlearn.net Toni Hager Neurodevelopment evaluations and home based programs.

Luke's Life List
www.joyceherzog.com Joyce Herzog Individualized Education Planner. Over 100 pages of life skills.

Multiplication and Division
Computer Program written by my husband Karl Kulp.

New Practice Readers
Phoenix Learning Resources. Graded readers for older students.

The Core Knowledge Series
E.D. Hirsch, Jr. *What Your 1st, 2nd, 3rd, 4th, 5th, 6th Grader* needs to know. Good education fundamentals.

Reading Works and Grammar Works
www.theworkspeople.com Multi-sensory step-by-step programs to teach writing, spelling, reading and grammar. Based on *The Writing Road to Reading* by Romalda Spalding.

Pathway Readers
Amish based readers that are black and white with easy to see text. Stories are wholesome - children are expected to obey and respect their parents and still have fun. Readers to 8th grade.

Math-U-See
www.mathusee.com Steve Demme Multi-sensory math program Build-Write-Say.

I Can Do It!
A micropedia of Living on Your Own. Marian B. Latzko. 1-888-357-7654. The best independent living guide-book I have found. Budgeting, finance. roommates, renting, eating right, cleaning, laundry and more!

Games for Learning
by Peggy Kaye. Peggy has also written *Games for Reading* and *Games for Math*.

Brain Builder®
Working Memory Skill Building. www.advancedbrain.com

Brain Gym®
Physical exercises that enhance brain function. Edu-Kinesthetics, Inc., www.braingym.com

Discover your child's desires
Lighting preference
  -low light
  -window light
  -no light
Temperature preference
  -open window
  -air conditioning
  -warm heat
Seating placement
Work
  -alone
  -with friend

More Ideas for teaching to processing differences

Visual	Auditory	Kinesthetic
Flashcards	Tapes	Dice and Cards
Pop-up books	Music	Clay
Slates	Oral reading	Games
Copy work	Educational videos	Computers
Board work	Computers	Construction
Diagrams	Direct teaching	Experiments
Workbooks	Songs	Manipulatives
Readers	Plays	Field trips
Magazines	Drama	Pop-up books
Letterwriting	Oral drills	Tactile flash cards
Storyboards	Interviews	Typing
Pantomime	Skip count	Writing in sand/air

and don't forget to laugh and dance and play . . .

FASD RESOURCES FOR FAMILIES

Overlapping Characteristics & Mental Health Diagnoses in Children

Cathy Bruer-Thompson

	FASD	ADHD/ADD	Sensory Int Dys	Autism	Bi-Polar	RAD	Depression	ODD	Trauma	Poverty
	Organic				Mood				Environ	
Easily distracted by extraneous stimuli	X	X	X	X						
Developmental Dysmaturity	X			X						
Feel Different from other people	X				X					
Often does not follow through on instructions	X	X					X	X	X	X
Often interrupts/intrudes	X	X	X	X	X		X			X
Often engages in activities without considering possible consequences	X	X	X	X	X					X
Often has difficulty organizing tasks & activities	X		X	X		X				X
Difficulty with transitions	X									
No impulse controls, acts hyperactive	X		X		X	X				
Sleep Disturbance	X				X		X		X	
Indiscriminately affectionate with strangers	X		X		X	X				
Lack of eye contact	X		X	X	X	X				
Not cuddly	X			X	X	X				
Lying about the obvious	X				X	X				
No impulse controls, acts hyperactive	X		X		X	X			X	
Learning lags: "Won't learn, some can't learn"	X		X				X		X	X
Incessant chatter, or abnormal speech patterns	X		X	X	X	X				
Increased startle response	X		X						X	
Emotionally volatile, often exhibit wide mood swings	X	X	X	X	X	X	X	X	X	
Depression develops, often in teen years	X	X					X		X	
Problems with social interactions	X			X	X		X			
Defect in speech and language, delays	X			X						
Over/under-responsive to stimuli	X	X	X	X						
Perseveration, inflexibility	X			X	X					
Escalation in response to stress	X		X	X	X		X		X	
Poor problem solving	X			X	X		X			
Difficulty seeing cause & effect	X			X						
Exceptional abilities in one area	X			X						
Guess at what "normal" is	X			X						
Lie when it would be easy to tell the truth	X				X	X				
Difficulty initiating, following through	X	X			X		X			
Difficulty with relationships	X		X	X	X	X				
Manage time poorly/lack of comprehension of time	X	X			X		X			X
Information processing difficulties speech/ language: receptive vs. expressive	X			X						
Often loses temper	X		X		X		X	X	X	
Often argues with adults	X				X			X		
Often actively defies or refuses to comply	X				X			X		
Often blames others for his or her mistakes	X	X			X		X	X		
Is often touchy or easily annoyed by others	X				X		X	X		
Is often angry and resentful	X						X	X		

Adapted from the work of Bruce Perry, Bessel van der Kolk, Diane Malbin, Minnesota Department of Education, Minnesota Department of Health, Ruby Payne

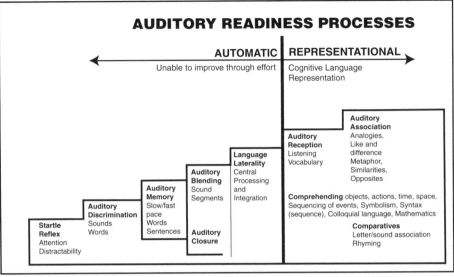

AUDITORY READINESS PROCESSES

AUTOMATIC — Unable to improve through effort

REPRESENTATIONAL — Cognitive Language Representation

Startle Reflex — Attention Distractability

Auditory Discrimination — Sounds, Words

Auditory Memory — Slow/fast pace, Words, Sentences

Auditory Blending — Sound Segments

Auditory Closure

Language Laterality — Central Processing and Integration

Auditory Reception — Listening, Vocabulary

Auditory Association — Analogies, Like and difference, Metaphor, Similarities, Opposites

Comprehending objects, actions, time, space, Sequencing of events, Symbolism, Syntax (sequence), Colloquial language, Mathematics

Comparatives — Letter/sound association, Rhyming

VISUAL READINESS PROCESSES

AUTOMATIC — Unable to improve through effort

REPRESENTATIONAL — Visual symbols and representations for Right and Left Cerebral Hemispheres

Light Reflex

Acuity Seeing — fine detail

Fixations — Saccadic Movements

Smooth Eye Pursuits — Motility, Horizontal, Vertical, Diagonal, Circle

Convergence and Fusion — Figure/ground, Simultaneous 3D vision, Depth perception

Visual Reception — Recognition of shapes, objects, focus, symbols, reading, pictures vocabulary, dot quality, directionality, silhouettes, matching and insets, closure

Visual Association Similarities — Like and difference, analogies, opposites, closure, grouping, classifying, patterns, relationships, directions (r,l) concepts

Visualization & Written Symbols — alphabet, words, numbers, phrase reading spelling, signs, visualization, 3D perspectives 3D drawings (solid and transparent) usable forms anticipate future, imagining past projecting (take another point of view)

Lyelle Palmer, Winona State University

How Can I Help My Child?

The 21st Century has been referred to as the century of the brain. We recommend that you research and utilize the best the world has to offer in training methods for top athletes, students and musicians.

You know your child - adapt accordingly.

"Culture defines who's 'disabled'. . . a child labeled dyslexic, hyperactive or learning-disabled in our society might excel in another culture."

Thomas Armstrong, *In Their Own Way,* J.P. Tarcher (1987).

"I am only one, but I am still one. I cannot do everything, but still I can do something. I will not refuse to do the something I can do."

Helen Keller

Helen Keller graduated with college honors in 1904, yet at age ten she was unble to see, hear or speak. By age 16 she had learned to read in Braille, speak and write well enough to attend college. Her teacher Anne Sullivan discovered the brain-body, mind-body connection because of her own struggles in learning.

Thank you Helen and Anne for your lights!

FASD RESOURCES FOR FAMILIES

What does neurodevelopment assesses:

Academic/Emotional: Where on the developmental scale is the child?

Auditory Perception: Does the child make sense of what she hears?

Spatial Awareness: Can the child make sense of what is outside herself? Is she aware of her body?

Body Integration: Can the child move in many directions? Can she wave her hands from one side of the body to the other (**midline crossing - horizontal & vertical**)?

Language: What it the listening level (**receptive language**)? How can the child communicate (**expressive language**)? What is the quality of the child's sounds (**articulation**)? Does the child have an inner voice dialogue or is all communication still external?

Memory: What level of short-term memory does the child have hearing (**auditory short term memory**) or seeing (**visual short term memory**)? What happens if you mix auditory and visual together?

Reflexive: What reflexes does the child have? Are the early infant reflexes still engaged?

Time, Sequence, Organization: (These skills are needed for classroom work.) What is the level of development of the child?

Visual Perception: Can the child look and understand what she sees, rather than just being able to see?

Visualization: Can the child make mental pictures?

"Be careful how you say things. You say concrete, I see pavement. I need things presented clear. Don't tell me my brain has holes like Swiss cheese. When you say Swiss cheese all I can think of is holes holes holes - I simply have a brain injury. It just doesn't connect right."

Delonzo, FASD, age 17

"How do I succeed with multiple children with FASD.

- *Predict what they are going to be doing.*
- *Provide the structure to keep them safe.*
- *Have eyes in the back of my head and tentacles into the community.*
- *A good sense of humor.*
- *Patience to teach and reteach.*
- *Reach out to other parents.*
- *Ability to parent by the seat of my pants.*
- *And a healthy dose of prayer.*

Ann Yurcek, FASD Mom
Author *Tiny Titan*

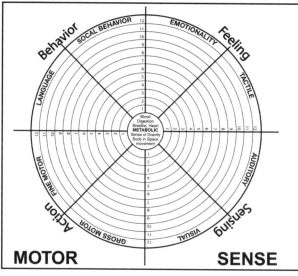

MOTOR **SENSE**

The Hager Nuerodevelopment Vortex

11-12	Integration
9-10	Frontal Cortex
8	Cortex
7	Cortex
6	Lower Cortex
5	Pre-Cortex
4	Upper Midbrain
3	Lower Midbrain
2	Pons
1	Medula

For more information regarding the
Hager Neurodevelopment Vortex visit
www.kidscanlearn.net

LIZ'S PROGRAM OUTLINE

We discovered when Liz mastered 75% of a lower level of development it was time to slowly introduce the next level. We offer this information in hopes we can provide you clues to help your child. Remember each child who has been prenatally exposed is different.

1. Unconditional love
2. Metabolic processing
- nutritional deficiencies
- chemical sensitivities
- allergies
- immune system functioning
- inflammation/infections
3. Reflexes
- muscle tone
- security in gravity
- sucking
- eye movement
- tactile defensiveness

4. Basic senses – Sensory input neurological *(each of the basic senses has its own develop ment sequence)*
- touch
- auditory
- visual
- balance **(vestibular)**
- kinesthetic
- body in space **(proprioception)**
5. Sensory-Integration
- touch
- auditory
- visual
6. Gross motor
- balance
- right from left
- motor planning
- visual motor integration
- knowing body's position
- use both sides of body
- dominance **(favor one side)**
7. Fine Motor
- use and control of mouth, tongue **(oral motor)**

- speech and language
- use and control of eyes **(ocular motor)**
- eye and hand coordination **(fingers)**
8. Body awareness
- attention
- concentration
- organization
- self-counsel
- visual perception
- visual motor planning
- visual motor integration
- concentration
- auditory perception
9. Detailing
- silent thinking
- writing
- reading
- math
- spelling
- imagination
- visualization
- interjection
- body language

INFORMATION ON FASD FOR FAMILIES AND FRIENDS
Parenting Ideas from Families in the Trenches

We need you! Children with brain injury need non-judgmental, loving friends and relatives who accept them as they are, encourage but not demand growth, and rejoice in strengths and accomplishments no matter how small.

What every child with FASD needs?

Unconditional love.

Acceptance.

Attention.

Supervision.

Patience and understanding.

Wisdom.

Structure / environmental controls.

Redirection.

Help to slow down when getting out of control (deceleration).

Someone who believes they are capable.

Ways to help our child grow

1. Praise their strengths.
2. Acknowledge their expression of frustration.
3. Respect their fears and difficulty with change.
4. Understand that behaviors may be a can't do it not a won't do it.
5. Talk to them as a person - not someone who is stupid.
6. Keep from comparing them with others.
7. Avoid joking, teasing or putting them down.
8. Refrain yourself from telling them, "you will grow out of this."
9. Get involved in their interests.
10. Find out what they are trying to learn and think of fun ways to join.

We need your help. It is exhausting to raise a child who has prenatal brain injury. Consider learning how to provide respite for us. Please understand this is a brain injury not an issue of 'bad' parenting and our child is not a 'bad' child.

We may have to avoid

- Holidays and birthdays
- Circus, concerts, movies, sport events
- These events may be too highly stimulating.

New people or visitors in our home are a change in routine and may be difficult for our child.

Things to remember

1. Poor impulse control is a brain injury issue and frustrating behaviors are most likley not intentional.
   - Keep your cool and refrain from yelling.
   - Why? Because the child is more than likely not misbehaving, but unable to understand certain things.
2. The child may not be able to do two things at once. For example: If you are eating or playing a game the child may not be able to talk.
3. The child may not be able to use their feet and hands at the same time.
4. View behavior problems as a disability that can be dealt with, rather than disobedience.
5. Think stretched toddler, our child may look like other children their age, but trust us when we tell you supervision issues, responsibility issues and amount of freedom. It is for your protection and our child's safety.

Tips on communicating with a child with FASD

1. Find a quiet place to talk. Why? Large, noisy busy areas are hard to communicate and function well in.
   a. Turn off radio or TV.
   b. Close door.
   c. Move to quieter area.

2. Began talking with simple topics.
    a. How is your dog?
    b. What did you eat for lunch?
3. Talk about things the child likes.
4. Stay on one topic.
5. State one sentence at a time.
    a. Make it easy for the child to participate in a conversation by asking yes and no questions.
    b. Remain still or walk at the same speed as the child when talking.
6. Keep sentences short.
7. Instead of asking why, use words like where, how, what, who or when. Why will send their brain in a house of mirrors.
8. Allow time for child to respond, refrain from hurrying child.
    a. If our child can not get the right word, don't fill in, give clues or description or ask the child to point.
    b. Repeat a point using different words Keep information simple.
9. Give them choices to ease decisionmaking, but still allow independence of choice.
10. Be an active listener.
    a. Give frequent eye contact.
    b. Look for gestures.
    c. If understanding is unclear, take a guess (are you talking about . . . Oh now I get it.)
11. Tell others if you learn better ways to talk with our child so all can benefit.
12. Avoid behavior which winds our child up. Such as tickling, wrestling and pillow fighting.
13. Sit or squat next to our child, do not stand over.
14. In a group, make sure the child is placed so conversation can be around them.
15. May not be able to express needs such as thirst, hunger, going to toilet and may fidget instead.

16. Look through the child's eyes.
    a. How we look at things or understand things may be totally different from how they understand something.
    b. Consider watching *Forrest Gump* with Tom Hanks to get an idea of concrete thinking.

EXAMPLES

"Embarrassed? No, I've never been embarrassed. Why would I be embarrassed?"
Because the child had a hot foot. a dirty tennis sho had just landed ten feet away, hitting an older woman on the back of the leg. His logic was that the person who was hit was dumb to be standing i the way.

"You can only buy something under $10."
An armload of clothes later, the teen assumes you will purchase all she has found as long as each is under $10.00

"I had checks, what do you mean I didn't have money."
After writing a $59.99 check for a pair of shoes even though the bank balance was under $12.00.

"It's not my fault! They should have stopped me the first time."
A child caught on camera stealing disposable camera's from a store. The third offense.

"What do you mean I can't drive without a license. I can drive without a license."
After 28th sentence for driving with suspended license.

"I'm not in the girl's room, I'm on the carpet!"
Young man caught in a girl's room.

MANAGE

ANGER Drink a cold glass of filtered water or suck on an all natural fruit popsicle. Mix up in a blender fruit, ice and yogurt smoothie, then make the rest into popsicles for anger emergencies.

TIME OUT A pup tent or large box filled with blankets, cuddle toy and/or pillows is a safe recluse to regain composure.

GAIN ATTENTION Clap hands to a beat. Clap one time if you hear me. Clap two times if you hear me. Clap three times if you hear me.

GAIN QUIET Speak in whisper, mouth words or turn down lights.

Life Stories and Role Play

Make up short nighttime behavior stories about a child learning to do something new you want your child to learn. Tell the story repeatedly and have your child begin to tell it as you practice new behavior.

Host dress rehearsals for starting school year, holidays, restaurants and birthday parties.

Faith-based Activities

Practice place of worship events before you go. Watch a television service, tape a service, practice being quiet, sitting and standing.

Provide a signal for the child to let you know they need to take a break. Show them the appropriate way to leave a service. . .practice when you are not in a service. Know the location of the bathroom.

Focus on communication, behavior modeling in small steps and good relationships. Your child will teach you more about Faith, Patience, Truth and Love than you ever imagined.

Think different birthdays

Birthdays can be very overwhelming:
• Let the child pick out their own presents and don't wrap them. The energy of the surprise may be hard for child to handle.
• Start the day with a special breakfast and a few tiny presents.
• Wear matching family T-shirts on holidays, community events and birthdays.
• If you host a party keep it organized and simple.
• Have the child pick their favorite dinner

Think different holidays and events

• New Year's Party on the child's time zone while they're still awake. Make a time capsule using a can with a lid. Write a New Years wish. Put a picture of the child, favorite toy, food, color, story. Open the capsule next New Year to see how much they have changed.
• Adopt a family for a holiday.
• Have a holiday tea party with the family - tea, cookies or appetizers
• Buffet dinners work better than pass the food. A large 3 sided box with a child table inside can provide a small separate room for children to dine in, a place for food to fall and quiet.
• Make a paper chain. The child can rip off a chain per day to count down to the holiday.
• Valentine's Day everyone in family says three nice thing about every other family member.
• Thanksgiving Trees from Nov. 1 to 31 secretly place paper leaves with notes of thanksgiving on a bare twig tree.
• Have a pajama day. Stay home, goof off and do things together.
• Develop a bedtime or wake up ritual.

Shopping

• Unless you need a person to help you when your child is having an instore meltdown - simply say - "My child is upset. We are practicing calming down when shopping techniques. Everything will be fine. She is doing much better today."

Controlled successes

Provide opportunities for your child to succeed.

• A carnival game that allows every child to win.

• Visit to the amusement park on Mother's Day when all the other mother's are doing something else and there are no crowds.

• Set an attainable goal and break into very small steps and show progress to a larger goal on a posted chart with stickers

• Enjoy short periods of time at an event and then leave to integrate child in community life

  • Circus to see the lions.
  • Sunday worship and leave before service.
  • Parade to see one marching band.
  • Museum to see dinosaurs.
  • Library to get one book.
  • Restaurant to have desert.
  • Grocery shopping to get less than ten things

Controlled failures

We allow our child to fail at times so that she/he learns the consequences. We offer Plan A and Plan B. Plan A allows the child to do it the way he chooses. Plan B provides another way to handle a situation. We role play both plans. We discovered 'real life' experiences provided better opportunity to make a permanent memory, so sometimes we allow him to try his way and fail. Once the choice is made, we provide the supports to help him learn from his choice.

RELAX

BATHE Epsom Salt Bath. Add 1 cup of epsom salt to a tub of water and soak. Shower after bathing.

BAROQUE MUSIC (Mozart, Handel, Bach, Vivaldi) Initial research in the 60's by Georgi Lazanov (Bulgarian Psychologist) and further scientific research has shown that a slow, relaxing tempo of one beat per second can sometimes affect memory recall and learning.

AROMATHERAPY Smell bypasses the thalamus region of the brainstem and connects directly with neurons in the cortex creating a direct route to our memory. Essential oils are highly concentrated and need to be used with care and applied 'only' by the drop. Grapeseed, almond or hazelnut oil are good carriers for them. Use in potpourri or in a tea kettle to scent a room, add to a candle or spray mister sprinkle on a tissue in a small plastic bag, add to bath water, unscented lotions or shampoos. Natural scents can be used as insect repellents or in laundry. **NIGHT MARE SPRAY:** Fill a spritz bottle with water and add a few drops of jasmine, lavender, chamomile or ylang-ylang. Let child spray away night time monsters and fears.

SLEEP A humidifier with jasmine, lavender, chamomile or ylang-ylang. When Liz has a cold we add eucalyptus. The humidifier makes it easier to breathe and also adds a soft white noise. Time in the sun, a day outside, a quiet evening, a hottub, sauna or bath, turning the lights down in your home an hour before bedtime, a medically certified magnet mattress, natural nutrients to encourage sleep (melatonin). Automatic timer on lights to turn them up an hour before waking time.